This book is dedicated to SISTER MARY LOUISE TIBEAU and to L.H. DEWEY,
two pioneers in the field of cannabis research.

Sugar Magnolia, sweet blossom blooming,
We can have high times if you'll abide
We can discover the wonders of nature
Laying in the willows down by the riverside.

"Sugar Magnolia," courtesy the Grateful Dead

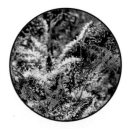

CONTENTS

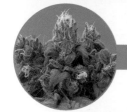
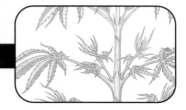
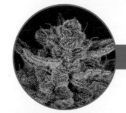
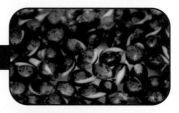
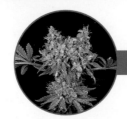
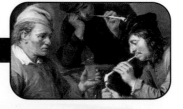

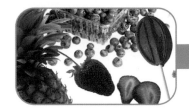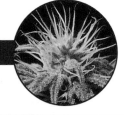
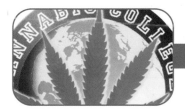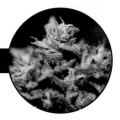
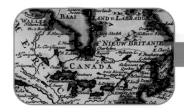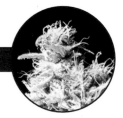
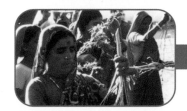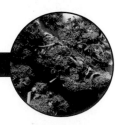

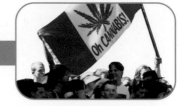
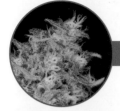
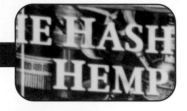
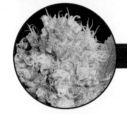
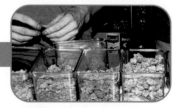
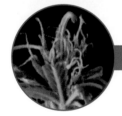
www.bigbookofbuds.com

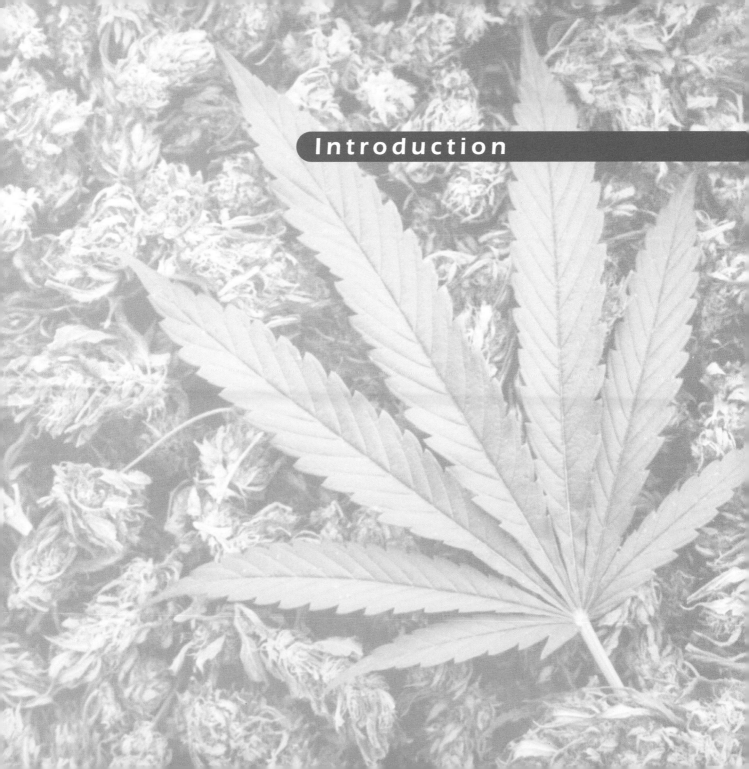

Introduction

An introduction is supposed to be a key that unlocks the method for using the information in the volume at hand. As a reader of the very first book to survey contemporary marijuana varieties, you deserve that help. I have been asked to provide it. However, before I begin, I would like to talk a little about the breeders, since this book celebrates their achievements.

Breeders are a breed apart. They are a different kind of people than you or me. They are egotistical, competitive, and driven by obsessions. If these people are so vain, why would we devote a book to their work? Doesn't it just encourage them? Yes. And that's exactly the point. Breeders must be tough, tenacious and thick-skinned in order to pursue their careers. Breeding is not easy. It requires a keen eye, an acute sense of taste and most important, an ability to discern a plant with outstanding potency. Not many people have this ability—a sort of perfect pitch in the area of THC and cannabis. In addition to skill, an inspired breeder has an intuitive ability to choose the right one. This book celebrates 100 right choices.

The Big Book of Buds also celebrates the success of the cannabis culture. Despite opposition from virtually every government around the world, marijuana and the cultures it has fostered have thrived. In the face of the "War on Drugs," an individualistic campaign to "overgrow the government" has stopped the campaign for a "Drug Free World." The companies featured here have all helped to tip the balance.

Seed breeders and their companies have socially redeeming values other than their resistance to various governments' campaigns of cultural genocide. They are the ones who help us change not what we think, but how we think it. From ruderalis type progenitors thousands of years ago, successions of breeders have coaxed and twisted the plant's genes into hemp and marijuana, sativas and indicas. Today's breeders are following a noble tradition of helping cannabis to adapt to new environments and to yield its precious products to humans.

While we celebrate the breeders and their creations, let's not forget our appreciation of this wondrous plant. Its decision to develop a synergistic relationship with an animal species—humans—has had an enormous effect on our development, as we have had on its fortunes. From its start in the Himalayan foothills, this plant has been carried all over the world, to every climate, by humans who have used it for many purposes. They have helped it fit into its new homes. In return, cannabis has helped societies progress time and time again, for thousands of years. The experience of the two species in the last 40 years has been just another turn in the spiral of their coexistence. Two things are certain as this story continues: These species will continue to travel together, and the journey will cover new areas of the spiral.

We can see the evolution from year to year. Twenty years ago there were only two seed companies, The Seed Bank and SSSC. The Seed Bank merged with Sensi Seeds more than a decade ago. An industry has bloomed since these pioneers ventured into the business. Public interest in different varieties is widespread.

It will soon be 4:20 somewhere in the world. Let's use this occasion to toast the breeders, past, present and future. Also to thank Cannabis, which allows itself to be twisted and turned in our dance of life.

Now let's move on to the serious work of a mini-lesson on how to use this book.

As you may have surmised from leafing through or checking the title, this is a book about buds. That might seem obvious, but it is more than just a book with dramatic photos and excellent design, fine for a coffee table or to be placed behind the glass of an heirloom display. It contains some very informative essays on seeds, varieties and cannabis history, as well as some insightful stories and anecdotes. It also offers useful information for any level of enthusiast on some of the most acclaimed marijuana varieties in the world.

Information on the varieties in this volume comes directly from the mouths of the breeders themselves. Varieties are arranged alphabetically for easy reference. One appendix in the back divides the varieties by company and another lists the critical information about the companies that the breeders represent.

Each variety page features quick reference icons that let you check certain characteristics at a glance. Allow me to introduce you to each icon and its uses.

The Icons

The first icon deals with plant type. The possibilities are:

(S) which represents plants with over 80% sativa background,

(I) with a background of 80% or more indica,

and hybrids, which are either

(SI) more sativa or

(IS) more indica.

(I) Indica plants originated around the 30th parallel in the Hindu Kush region of the Himalayan foothills. This includes the countries of Afghanistan, Pakistan, Tajikistan, Northern India and Nepal. The weather there is quite variable from year to year. For this reason, the populations there have a varied gene pool and even within a particular population there is a high degree of heterogeneity, which results in plants of the same variety having quite a bit of variability. This helps the population survive. No matter what the weather during a particular year, some plants will survive and reproduce.

These plants are fairly short, usually under 5 feet tall. They are bushy with compact branching and short internodes. They range in shape from a rounded bush to a pine-like shape with a wide base. The leaves are short, very wide and a darker shade of green than most equatorial sativas because they contain larger amounts of chlorophyll. Sometimes there is webbing between the leaflets. At the 30th latitude, the plants don't receive as much light as plants at or near the equator. By increasing the amount of chlorophyll, the cells use light more efficiently.

Indica buds are dense and tight. They form several shapes depending on variety. All of them are chunky or blocky. Sometimes they form continuous clusters along the stem. They have intense smells ranging from acrid, skunky, or musky to equally pungent aromas. Indica smoke is dense, lung-expanding and cough-inducing. The high is heavy, body-oriented and lethargic.

(S) Sativa plants grow between the equator and the 50th parallel. They include both marijuana and hemp varieties. The plants that marijuana growers are interested in come from the equator, between the 20th parallel North and South. Countries from this area are noted for high-grade marijuana include Colombia, Jamaica, Nigeria, Congo, Thailand, and Sumatra. Populations of plants from most of these areas are quite uniform for several reasons. Cannabis is not native to these areas. It was imported to grow hemp crops and then it adapted over many generations, with human intervention. Each population originated from a small amount of fairly uniform seeds from the region between the 45th and 50th parallels. Then the populations evolved over hundreds of generations with the help of humans. This led to fairly uniform populations in climates that vary little from year to year.

Sativas grow into 5-15 feet tall, symmetrical pine-shaped plants. The space between the leaves on the stem, the internode, is longer on sativas than indicas. This helps to give sativas a taller stature. The lowest branches are the widest, spreading $1\frac{1}{2}$ to 3 feet. Because the branches grow opposite each other, plant diameters may reach 6 feet. The leaves are long, slender and finger-like. The plants are light green since they contain less chlorophyll.

Sativa buds are not as dense as indica buds. Some varieties grow buds along the entire branch, developing a thin, compact cola. Others grow large formations of very light buds. The smoke is sweet, spicy or fruity. The highs are described as soaring, psychedelic, thoughtful and spacy.

IS Indica-sativa hybrids naturally tend toward the indica side of the family. They usually have controlled height. They don't grow very tall and after forcing flowering, their growth is limited. Their side branches are usually not prominent and they can be grown in a small space.

SI Sativa-indica hybrids tend toward the sativa parentage. They are taller plants, and will grow to double or triple their size if they are forced when they are small. They are usually hard to grow in a sea of green, as the plants demand more space to spread out.

With the many combinations and complex parentages of modern hybrids, it is impossible to generalize about the qualities of hybrids' smoke, high or other characteristics. So many plants have been crossed and their progeny used for breeding that it is truly a mixed-up world out there. *The Big Book of Buds* will answer your questions regarding characteristics of particular varieties.

The second icon details the number of days it takes the plant to ripen after forcing flowering. Both environmental conditions and subjective factors affect maturation.

Take, for instance, one experiment in which identical plants grown indoors in a lab were fed different water-soluble commercial fertilizers. These identical plants, grown with identical conditions except the fertilizers, ripened up to 10 days apart. The fertilizers also affected the taste and quality of the buds.

Plant growth and maturation is also affected by temperature. Both cold and hot conditions interfere with ripening. Temperate conditions encourage fast growth and prompt ripening.

The planting method is another factor that affects ripening time. Hydroponic plants mature earlier than their sisters in planting media.

I would call a plant ripe when the "resin" in the glands starts to turn milky or amber. This is about a week later than some people prefer. The taste differs and the cannabinoids may change a bit, resulting in different highs. Dutch coffeeshops often sell bud that is immature. The glands are there, but have not filled completely with THC. The high is racing and buzzy. I don't find it very satisfying. Obviously, ripening time is affected by your idea of ripeness.

It is easy to see that the numbers mentioned are intended to give the reader approximations rather than hard figures. While they offer indications of what you should expect, they shouldn't be used as the sole source to figure your timetable.

Plants that are recommended for growing outdoors indicate the maturity date under natural light. When no latitude is mentioned, figure the month indicated is at the same latitude as the country of origin. For Holland, the latitude is 52 degrees. Canadian seeds are produced at 50 degrees latitude and Swiss seeds are produced at 47 degrees latitude.

The third icon indicates recommendations for planting. The choices are:

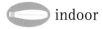 indoor   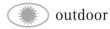 outdoor

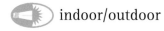 indoor/outdoor

Outdoor strains may do well in a greenhouse set-up, but will be difficult to grow indoors. They may require too much light for inside growing, and usually have their own ideas about growth and height, making them hard to tame. The problem with most plants not recommended for outdoors in temperate climates is that the plants don't ripen by the end of the season. Some plants rated as indoor plants can be grown outdoors if they are forced to flower early using shade cloth. As an example, a plant that ripens in mid-November, 45 days after a gardener's September 30th harvest schedule, could be coaxed to flower early by covering it with opaque plastic each evening at 6 pm and removing it at 6 am the next morning, beginning July 1 and continuing through late August. Most varieties will ripen within 75 days.

The fourth icon reports the expected yield. These figures are somewhat ambiguous because results are not reported consistently. Cannabis, like all green plants, uses light to fuel photosynthesis. The sugars produced become tissue. As a shortcut, you could say Light=Growth. Yields vary first and foremost due to light conditions, so space or plant definitions are incomplete by themselves. The yields suggested here assume that indoor gardens are receiving at least 600 watts per meter (wpm) where no light wattage is indicated.

SOG The fifth icon is listed only when plants are suitable for sea of green gardens. Plants in these gardens are spaced together very closely so that each plant needs to grow little if any to fill the canopy. Plants are forced to flower soon after they are placed in the flowering space. Eliminating the vegetative growth stage decreases turnaround. SOG gardens hold 3 to 6 plants per square foot (30-60 plants per meter^2).

The sixth icon offers the parentage of the variety. While this can get quite complex, you get an idea of what the possibilities are for any variety by knowing its parents.

Some of the hybrids in the book are f2 unstabilized. When pure strains (let's call them strains A and B) are crossed and a hybrid is produced, the first generation, the f1 hybrid plants, are all uniform because they all contain the same genes, one set from the female and one set from the male. When two f1s are crossed, the seeds receive a random assortment of genes. For each of the more than 100,000 sets of genes, a plant may get two genes from A one each from A and B or two from B. No two plants are alike.

To stabilize them so that they have similar characteristics, the plants are inbred for 5 or 6 generations creating an f6, using careful selections. Breeders often work with unstabilized hybrids, which has an advantage when breeding for cloning.

Stability can be judged in part by the number of parents a variety has. Pure strains are the most uniform, since they are not recombining different genetic dispositions. Hybrids have the advantage of gaining vigor from the fresh combination. They also vary more. Strains with 3 or 4 parents are likely to exhibit more than one phenotype when grown out. When multiple parents are hybrids themselves, the combination can result in quite a bit of diversity.

Diversity is not always bad. Consider a gardener starting out. Clones are taken once the plants grow some side stems. When the plants have been harvested and tasted, the gardener decides to select two plants for the next garden. Clones of those plants are grown vegetatively and used for mothers. If the seed line is uniform, as it is with pure strains or stabilized varieties, there will not be much difference between the plants. Seeds from an unstabilized variety give the gardener more choices.

The seventh icon is the one that is most important to me. What is the high like? Describing a state of mind is not an easy task. Separating one's mental state from the state of mind created by the brain in interplay with cannabinoids is subtle. We have used many terms to describe the buzz:

alert ▪ body stone ▪ cerebral ▪ cheerful ▪ clear head ▪ couch lock ▪ creative ▪ creeper ▪ energetic ▪ euphoric ▪ even body-head high ▪ giggly ▪ happy ▪ lethargic ▪ mellowing ▪ munchies ▪ narcotic ▪ physically relaxing ▪ psychedelic ▪ sleepy ▪ social ▪ stoney ▪ trippy ▪ uplifting ▪ visual ▪ wandering mind

The eighth icon, the final one, is a short, 1 to 3 word description of the smell and taste. The odors are:

acrid ▪ ammonia ▪ berry ▪ bubblegum ▪ citrus ▪ dry ▪ earthy ▪ floral ▪ fresh ▪ fruity ▪ hashy ▪ chocolate ▪ mango ▪ melon ▪ musky ▪ old sock ▪ peppery ▪ pineapple ▪ piney ▪ pungent ▪ skunk ▪ smooth ▪ spicy ▪ sandalwood ▪ sweet ▪ tart ▪ tobacco ▪ tropical ▪ woodsy

Fuller descriptions of the buzz, taste and smell are found in the text. You will also find DJ Short's palate chart of odor and taste on p. 53 most informative.

The icons are fast reference points. They give you an idea of where the story is going. The text accompanying each variety fleshes out this information with more nuanced descriptions and tips about the plant's preferences. Every variety offers something a little different.

The stories are engaging. Still, we have to admit that the photos are the most engaging part. They show what words can only suggest. Some of the pictures almost take you inside the bud. I'm sure they will provide you with hours of sightseeing pleasure.

Enjoy the book. Next time we'll try to make it scratch and sniff. Or even better, scratch and inhale.

Quick Key to Icons

Sensory Experience

 Buzz   Taste/Smell

Strain Type

 Sativa   Indica   Sativa/Indica   Indica/Sativa

Growing Info

 Flowering Time   Indoor 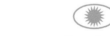 Outdoor   Indoor/ Outdoor

 Parents   Yield   Sea of Green

Breeder Location

 South Africa   Australia   Canada   Netherlands   Switzerland

Varieties

AK-47

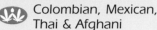

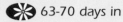 65/35

 63-70 days in

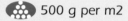 500 g per m2

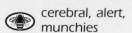 Colombian, Mexican, Thai & Afghani

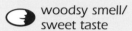 cerebral, alert, munchies

woodsy smell/ sweet taste

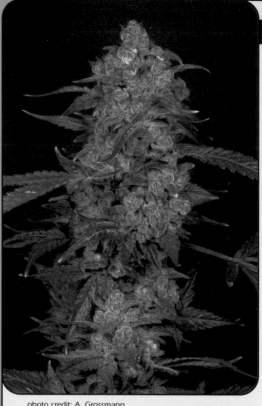

photo credit: A. Grossmann

Despite its aggressive name, AK-47 has many peaceful tendencies. First bred in 1992, the name suggests the power packed in its dark, resinous, compact buds that bristle with red hairs and glistening trichomes. AK-47 has a spiced aroma bordering on skunk, with a hint of sandalwood, but tastes sweeter and more floral than the smell would lead one to expect.

AK has mostly sativa characteristics with one exception: a quick finishing time. This variety was reworked in 1999 to increase stability, so results from seeds are uniform. A tall plant with substantial girth and big fat calyxes, she performs excellently in indoor environments, both soil and hydro, and has been grown outdoors with good results in Spain. In low to medium temperatures this variety produces a denser bud; in high temperatures buds are fluffier and more open, but total yields are roughly equivalent.

The AK-47 buzz is immediate and long lasting with an alert but mellow cerebral effect. Lab tests have rated the THC content at over 20 percent, making it a "one hit wonder" for many smokers. This variety can be a little spacey, but is great for playing and listening to music, or other social activities with friends. AK-47 helped put Serious Seeds on the map with a 2nd place finish in the hydroponics competition and a 3rd place in the overall category at the 1995 Cannabis Cup in the Netherlands. Overall, AK-47 has won 7 awards.

I

 42-50 days

 in preferred

 soil: 1 oz per plant
hydro: 2 oz per plant

 Skunk & Northern Lights

 sleepy, couch lock

light skunk

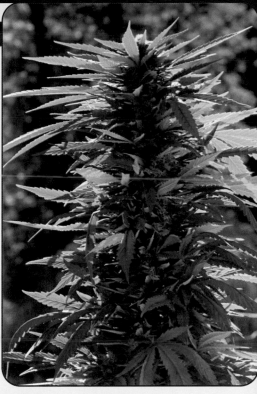

Americano received its name because this variety was selected specifically for Americans who came up to Vancouver looking for bulk marijuana. Traits that appealed to this market were the basis for selection, including a crystallized appearance with a lack of red or orange hairs, and tight buds that fill a pound bag well. This all-indica plant is a hybrid stabilized from the best outdoor and indoor indica strains grown by Enterprise Seed breeders.

The Americano high is a trademark indica buzz that will land you on the couch for a while, maybe encourage some napping. The taste is in the Skunk family, but pleasantly scented rather than overwhelmingly dank.

Americano is best suited to indoor growing methods, especially using a rockwool hydroponic or an aeroponic system. Indicas are known to have short growth cycles and this one does not disappoint with its shortest cycle finishing in as few as 6 weeks.

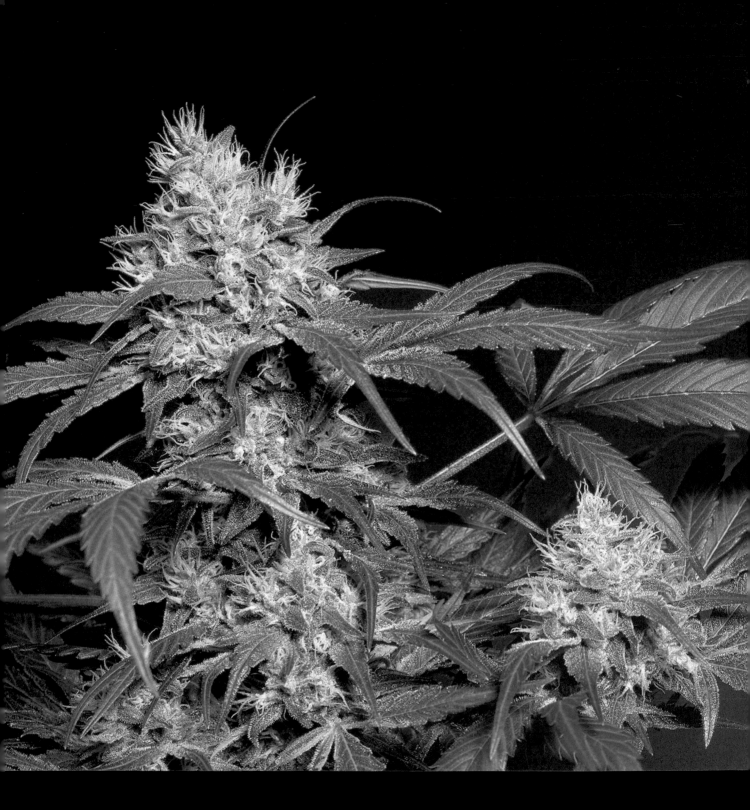

Amsterdam Flame

 I

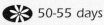 50-55 days

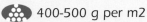 400-500 g per m2

 strains from India & California

 body relaxation

 fruit

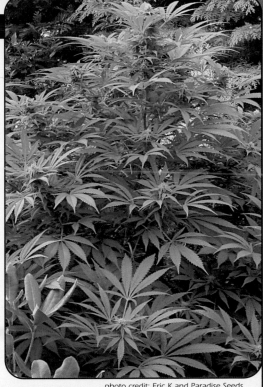

photo credit: Eric K and Paradise Seeds

Amsterdam Flame is a small-statured indica with colorful hairs ranging from the light orange that licks at the fire's edge to the incandescent violet of the flame's center. Foliage surrounding the bud is highly crystallized and dewy with resin, making this plant primo for hash lovers.

The mostly indica genetics mean that she is a bit bushy, with big fan leaves, and she doesn't stretch much indoors. Her structure is Christmas-tree-like, requiring a little more space in a sea of green setting. The controlled size does not take away from an impressive yield, typically with one main huge bud, requiring fewer plants to produce good harvests. Indoors, the Flame does well in hydro, coco or soil media. Outside she can overcome her petite nature to grow over 6 feet (2 meters) tall, and branch out to be 6 feet wide. In a good season at temperate outdoor latitudes, a plant of these proportions can yield a half-kilo or more per plant.

With a THC content at 19.2 percent, this variety produces a pleasantly potent high. Amsterdam Flame combines bodily relaxation with a sweet fruity smell in the mango family to create a truly outstanding gourmet bud that satisfies all the senses. The taste is soft and subtle with a hint of strawberry. Potentially a sleeper, Amsterdam Flame is more inclined to a euphoric ease, with a body sensation like a marijuana massage. Bred in 1994 by Paradise Seeds, Amsterdam Flame has gained popularity in Germany and Austria.

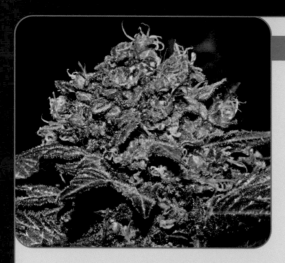

Atomic Northern Lights

 IS 65/35

  50-65 days in mid-Oct out

100 g per plant in 400 g per plant out

stable hybrids from Holland & Northwest U.S.

even head-body

sweet and pungent

SOG

Atomic Northern Lights has a history that spans continents. Afghani indica seeds were brought to the Northwest U.S. in the 1980s, then crossed with a Thai Haze and stabilized indoors because of the rainy, inhospitable weather. After a stint in the Northwest U.S., this variety ventured to Holland, where it continued to be developed and stabilized by Sensi as the notorious, award-winning Northern Lights. Seeds from this three-time Cannabis Cup winner were brought back to Canada by Dr. Atomic, who hybridized it with distant relatives of the same variety that had never made the overseas voyage. Dr. Atomic reunited these distant relations, separated by continents for generations, creating a vigorous new strain that diversified the Northern Lights genetic source.

Atomic Northern Lights shows its indica heritage in its growth characteristics, producing a short stocky plant that has a relatively quick flowering time. The buzz has a wider bandwidth than the typical indica-dominant variety, providing a balanced mind and body high that has an overall uplifting effect. Atomic Northern Lights is a smooth smoke with a sweet pungent flavor.

This classic, evergreen-tree-shaped plant is not too branchy and works well as "pole pot," staked with one center cola and up to four side colas that are smaller. If trimmed properly, Atomic Northern Lights works well in a sea of green. Dr. Atomic prefers soil growing methods, but this hardy plant will give satisfying results in most gardening set-ups.

This microscopic view reveals the structure of marijuana's treasured trichomes. These stalked glands have a stem and a ball-like tip that resembles a mushroom. The balled tip, balanced atop the stalk, contains THC. Growers, breeders and cannabis connoisseurs value the presence of a resinous sheen—that lustrous sparkle that is more than frosting: It's the magic ingredient of marijuana's potency.

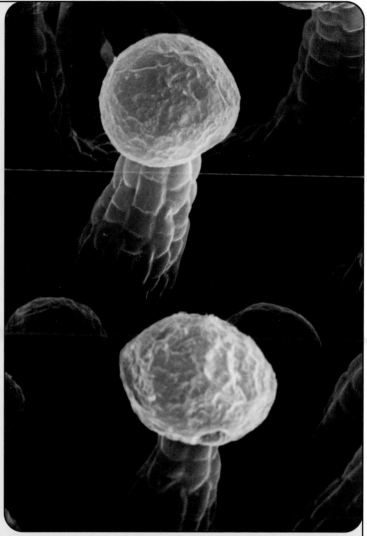

Trichome (stalked gland) of female plant.
photo credit: Dr. Paul Mahlberg

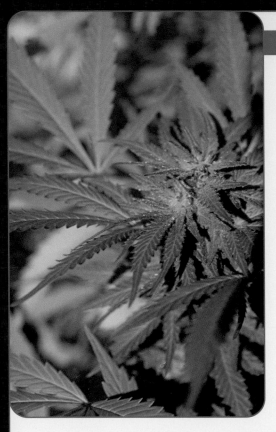

Bahia Black Head

 70/30

 early to mid-Aug

 1.5 kilo per plant

 Pure Brazil x KC 606 (m) x KC 606(m)

 sleepy, body high, munchies

 hashy

Bahia Black Head originated in 1998 with a pure Brazilian strain from a friend in Rio de Janeiro that was then crossed with a KC male. The cross produced a variety with the exquisite qualities of the Brazilian sativa intact, but with an earlier finishing time better for temperate zones.

As a mostly indica plant, Bahia Black Head is bushy, with leaves that are very bright in the beginning. The leaves and bud both turn a very deep dark green as she matures. As the plant grows, the new leaves are smaller, revealing a hint of sativa heritage. The buds tend to be an advantageous medium size that resist mold and moisture well.

Bahia Black Head has a distinctly Brazilian flavor that is strong and slightly hashy, as is the smell. The buzz is a heavy indica stone that may encourage some quality couch time, although munchie motivation may set you in motion.

KC Brains offers some plants that are especially intended for outdoors, where they are allowed to grow large. Bahia Black Head has the great advantage of an early finishing time for growers in temperate climes, but may require some work to remain clandestine: when allowed to grow outdoors for a full season, Bahia can get as tall as $6\frac{1}{2}$ feet (2 meters).

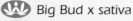

BC Big Bud

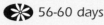 65/35

 56-60 days

 3-7 oz per plant in; up to 1lb per plant out

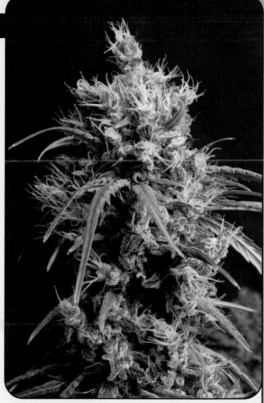 Big Bud x sativa

even head–body

citrus

SOG

photo credit: Barge

This British Colombian cousin to Big Bud will not disappoint. True to its name, it produces beautiful big buds that have a citrusy scent and flavor. While Big Bud from the Netherlands is mostly indica, BC Big Bud has been stabilized after a sativa cross. Its leaves are more sativa-like and the smoke has an enjoyable, cerebral high.

The resin production is outstanding, making crystal gems of the buds, and carpeting the leaves with dew drops. Even Big Bud's seeds are large, although seed size does not necessarily correspond to eventual plant or bud outcome.

This variety can be grown indoors or out, but due to large solid buds, care should be taken to avoid overmoisture as this could encourage mold. Indoors, it is happy in a hydroponic set-up and can be used in a sea of green method, or allowed to grow large with multiple branching.

T his illustration by **K. Abellán** deconstructs the mysterious botany of the cannabis plant from seed to maturity. The lingo for marijuana's botanical components are sometimes familiar and sometimes strangely scientific. A truly amazing plant, cannabis is the only known dioecious (gendered) annual in the plant kingdom.

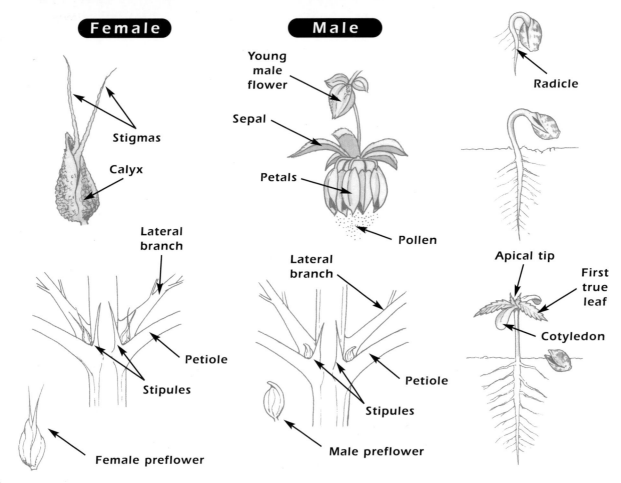

Female

Stigmas

Calyx

Lateral branch

Petiole

Stipules

Female preflower

Male

Young male flower

Sepal

Petals

Pollen

Lateral branch

Petiole

Stipules

Male preflower

Radicle

Apical tip

First true leaf

Cotyledon

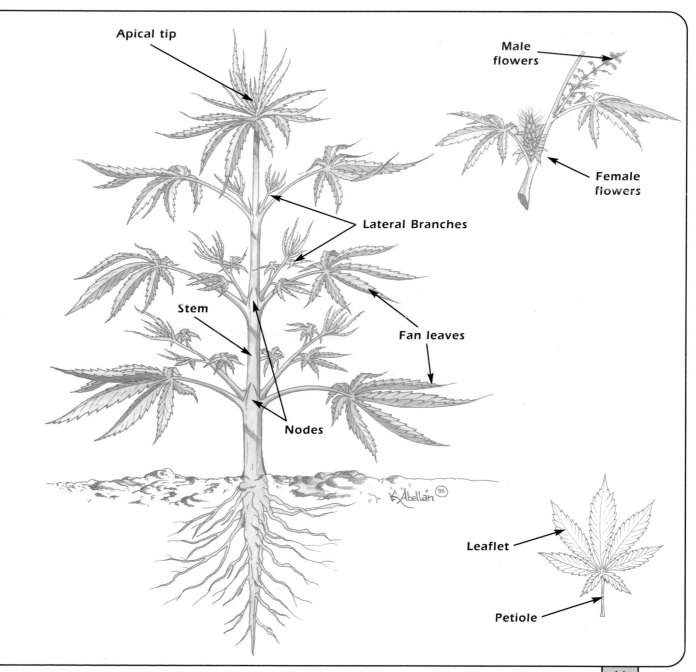

Apical tip

Male flowers

Female flowers

Lateral Branches

Stem

Fan leaves

Nodes

Leaflet

Petiole

Belladonna

60 days

450-500 g per m2 in; up to 600 g per plant out

 Super Skunk & mostly sativa (m)

trippy

fruity and pungent

SOG

Mostly sativa with indica tendencies, Belladonna is an ideal cross for quality and yield. Paradise Seeds introduced this variety in 1999, and since that time it has gained interest with commercial growers.

This variety combines a quick harvest time with a sativa high. In part named for her beauty, Belladonna is a pleasant looking plant with moderate foliage, indica growth patterns and tight, slightly orange buds. The aroma is fruity and pungent, and the taste is also fruity with some spice. Belladonna delivers a trippy high with peaks of hallucinogenic rushes.

No prima donna, Belladonna thrives in all environments. While popular in California and Spain, she has performed well outdoors even in the less hospitable Dutch climate. Her resistance to mold may be in part responsible for her outdoor stamina. Indoors, she does well in a sea of green set-up. Using this method, flowering can begin as soon as the plants are 6 inches (15 cm) tall, because they will continue to grow in the flowering cycle to 2.5-2.75 feet (75-85 cm). Belladonna is not very bushy, making it possible to grow plants close together.

photo credit: Ed B. and Paradise Seeds

Betazoid

 60-65 days

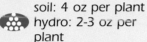

soil: 4 oz per plant
hydro: 2-3 oz per plant

Grapefruit, Northern Lights & African sativa

cerebral

fruity scent/ hashy taste

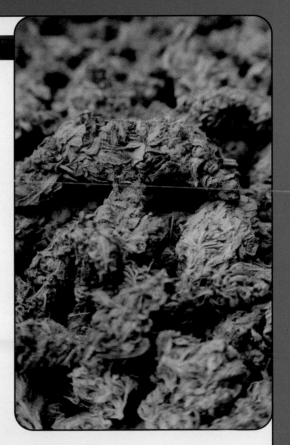

Help control your life . . .
realize your hidden potential . . .
counsel your doubts.
Strengthen your resolution and endurance . . .
release your pain.

This variety was bred and named Betazoid because it helped a friend kick a hard drug habit. With an alert, cerebral high typical of a sativa, Betazoid is considered to have characteristics beneficial to medical marijuana users, specifically those trying to maintain a positive frame of mind and alleviate chronic pain.

Betazoid was developed by selecting the best plants in a home set-up over three years of breeding. Selection was made again after the first generation was grown out and tested. The second selection was based on the quality of the high, the yield, the density of the nugs and the smoothness of the smoke. This strain has sturdy stems with bushy foliage and big tight buds that carry a mildly fruity scent. The flavor of the smoke has a deep hashish flavor.

This variety prefers to be cultivated in an indoor garden, and likes soil better than hydroponic set-ups. It will usually increase in size by ninety percent from the size at which it was flowered. Betazoid should only be grown outdoors in a temperate climate, with a finishing time of late September.

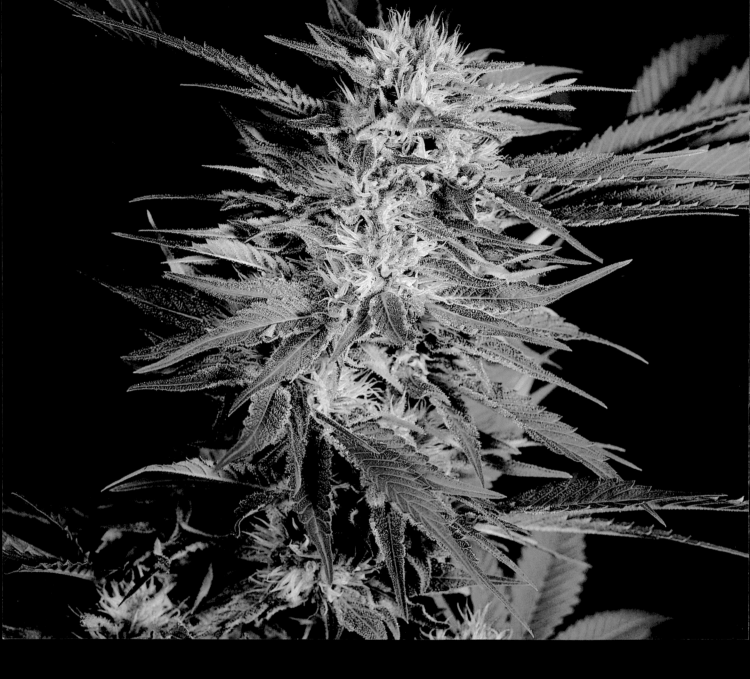

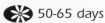

Big Bud

 50-65 days

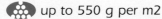

up to 550 g per m2

 SA a x BB x Skunk 18.5 (Afghani)

 body relaxation

 sweet and spicy

SOG

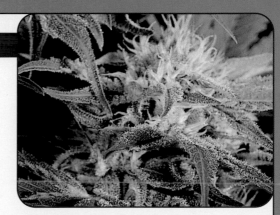

Big Bud is a classic favorite, and with good reason. This plant has traits that so many marijuana growers and enthusiasts are after: prodigious growth and a desirable high. Already a part of the Seed Bank breeding program in the 1980s, Big Bud was first sold as a hybrid with Skunk #1 from the Sacred Seed Company. This is the version that claimed the 1989 win in the mostly indica category at the Cannabis Cup. In the 1990s, Sensi Seeds and the Seed Bank merged and new attention was given to this hybrid. Another sweet, high-yielding, heavily indica line was crossed into the original hybrid, making this plant-type sweeter and more delicious to connoisseurs. With the new burst of flavor, the strain became interesting for more than just its heavy yields, which resulted in a fully unexpected prize for Big Bud in the 1996 Cannabis Cup.

As the name suggests, this variety is a producer: it is a good idea to tie up bottom branches because they may break due to the weight. A large internode ratio means that this variety requires minimal pruning to get maximum light to the flowers and makes an easy job of manicuring at harvest. Big Bud is fairly short with a traditional indica leaf structure, but unlike the stereotypical indica, can become tall and lanky if not closely tended. As with the typical indica/sativa hybrid, Big Bud may triple in size from the time the light cycle is changed. Big Bud also finishes in as few as 50 days with an impressive yield. The high is mellow with a sweet and spicy flavor, a long duration and a more indica body stone.

This variety is suitable for a sea of green method or for a garden of bigger plants. While relatively flexible, Big Bud has shown some sensitivity to the typical marijuana insects and pests. Best results occur in the indoor environment, where variables are more easily controlled. Hydro gives the best yields, but Big Bud can also thrive in soil, especially in the right outdoor conditions (not the case with the Netherlands weather). She can be expected to give the grower some beautiful flowers as long as they keep a tidy garden.

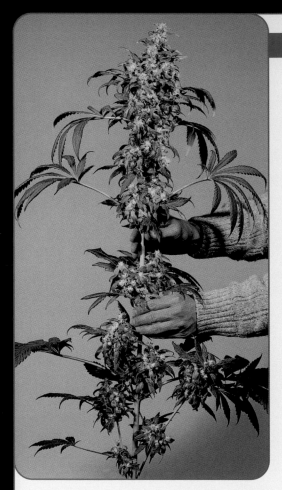

Black Domina

❄ 50 days

🌿 Afghani x Ortega 6 x Hash Plant

🐝 body relaxation, sleepy

up to 430 g per m2

acrid, hashy, peppery

SOG

Black Domina is a powerful smoke. Her resinous buds range from a harsh peppery scent to the dark smell of blackberries. Not intended for the sweet tooth, Black Domina buds taste smoky and spicy, leaving some tokers wondering if the pipe contains hashish along with the weed. She embodies the indica high, with overpowering body effects. While possibly devastating if used in the wrong circumstances, this strain is a great buzz for a day off or a nightcap when no serious work lies ahead.

This multiple cross is basically the result of stacking four of Sensi's heaviest selected indicas in one hybrid: the Afghani SA, the Ortega hybrid developed in Canada, and a combination of the Hash Plant and the famed Northern Lights, both of which have origins in the U.S. Pacific Northwest. Because 4-way hybrids are hard to stabilize, expect the f1 hybrid to show some variation—but also expect 90 percent of your plants to drip with resin.

The Black Domina plant has large bracts and wide-fingered, indica-style leaves. This variety was intended for indoor cultivation, and boasts a flower finishing time of under 2 months. The sea of green method is appropriate, but Black Domina will also be good as bigger, multibranched plants. If attempted outdoors, she may tend to run or produce lesser quality buds if the conditions are less than optimal. Growers at Sensi's Cannabis Castle recommend hydroponics for a clean and easy grow with the quickest and best results.

Black Widow

 50-70 days in mid-Oct out

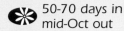

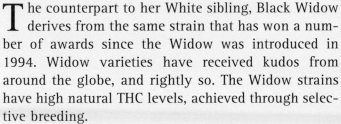 350-450 g per m2

 Brazilian sativa & South Indian hybrid

 clear, body relaxation

 pungent/ammonia with piney hues

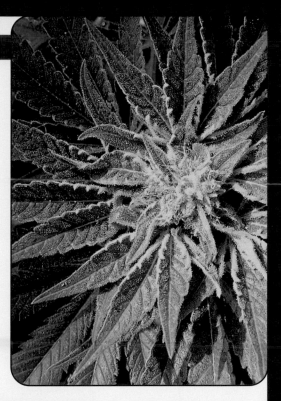

The counterpart to her White sibling, Black Widow derives from the same strain that has won a number of awards since the Widow was introduced in 1994. Widow varieties have received kudos from around the globe, and rightly so. The Widow strains have high natural THC levels, achieved through selective breeding.

Black Widow parted from her famous sister to follow her own color and genetic destiny with the establishment of Mr. Nice Seed Bank. She maintains the resin production that gives this variety a white, cobwebbed look. Her name has encompassed the added intrigue of the infamous female spider who devours her mate. Black Widow has a pungent, sweet scent with an acrid, ammonia overlay. The smoke's flavor improves upon the scent, tasting of sweet pine. The high is very lucid, but may sometimes make you want to lie in a hammock and doze.

This plant's structure is like a lanky Christmas tree. Black Widow likes TLC to achieve optimum results. For indoor methods, 8 to 10 weeks of flowering are necessary to produce the immense resin of which this plant is capable. In outdoor gardens, high rainfall can result in reduced yield. Great to use in experimental strains for the layman, the male pollen is recommended to achieve some interesting hybrids.

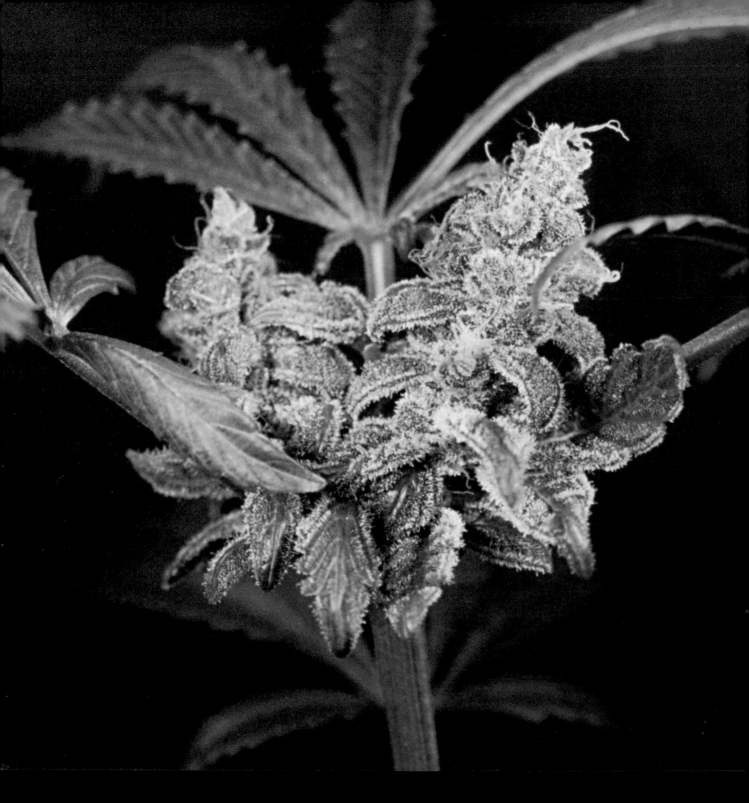

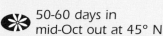
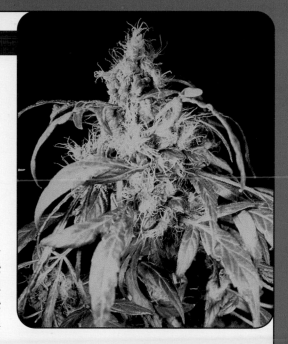

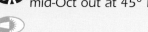 80/20

50-60 days in
mid-Oct out at 45° N

25 g per f2 with
40 wpf in; 300 g
per plant out

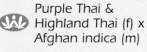 Purple Thai &
Highland Thai (f) x
Afghan indica (m)

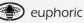 euphoric

berry of course

SOG

While Blueberry is a sativa/indica mix, it is subjectively considered a mostly indica cross. The name is obviously related to the flavor of the finished product, but also fits with the cool blue hues of the plant and buds, which will pale to a lavender blue in the curing and drying process.

Blueberry is a low to medium height plant of mostly indica structure, but with more branching, especially from the lower limbs. The plant grows full with wide, dark leaves and stems. Growing outdoors with organic fertilizers is optimal, as this allows Blueberry to retain the nuance of its flavors, making the quality utmost. This variety also performs well in terms of quality and quantity under many conditions, including the sea of green method.

The taste and aroma are very fruity, with the signature blueberry taste. This variety produces a notable and pleasantly euphoric experience of top quality, and the buzz lasts a long time. Blueberry smoke will not put you to sleep, but it may make you forget what you were going to do instead. Blueberry won first and second place for a number of *Cannabis Culture* "mini-Cups" sponsored by Marc Emery and *Cannabis Culture* magazine. Dutch Passion's version of Blueberry, which was derived from the original Delta 9 Collection, won first place in the 2000 *High Times* Cannabis Cup in the mostly indica category.

DJ Short on the Blue Family:

"The "Blue Family" of the herbal community originated from crosses of four varieties: Highland Thai, Chocolate Thai, Highland Oaxaca Gold, and Afghan Indica. All were pure P-1 contributing ancestors. Both Thai varieties and the Oaxaca were pure, land-race sativas. The seeds were gleaned from the connoisseur's choice herb of the late 1970s/early 1980s directly from their region of origin. The indica line came one generation removed from its region of origin in the mountains of Afghanistan and Pakistan via the growing community and network in Northern California and Southern Oregon.

The Highland Thai, also known as "Juicy Fruit Thai," produced a maze of many branches in a full, bushy tangle that was quite asymmetric, developing no easily identifiable main stem at maturity. The Oaxaca Gold was crossed with the Chocolate Thai to produce a plant that became known as "Purple Thai." The Purple Thai had symmetric branching patterns and grew tall with support. Both the Highland Thai and the Purple Thai were late bloomers, with finishing times that ranged between 10–16 weeks indoors or as late as mid-November outside, and sported at least minimal hermaphroditism. They each also produced champion herb that had little or no "ceiling" to them; that is, the more one consumed, the higher the experience.

The Purple and Highland Thai became the two female contributors to the Blue Family. Females were selected for overall quality of the finished product, including bouquet, flavor and buzz, as well as the lowest incidence of hermaphroditism. The Afghani Indica supplied the male P-1 pollen source. Selection among the Afghani plants was based on stout full structure and strong, musky, "skunkish" odor. The resulting cross grew very uniformly to a medium height, producing long, spear-shaped buds. I referred to this f1 simply as "the Cross." When two of these "Cross" plants were bred together, the resulting f2 "Double Cross" produced an extreme variation in phenotypic expression. It was from these varied Double Cross f2s that the Blue Family members were chosen and stabilized through several generations of selective breeding.

Blueberry x Nice

49 days

30 g per plant

 Blueberry (m) x Mr. Nice (f)

 up

 sweet and spicy

SOG

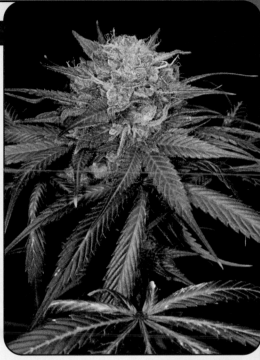

photo credit: Barge

The Blueberry x Nice hybrid has retained the poker straight structure of its mama, with minimal branching that makes sea of green gardening an easy method of choice. The sparing foliage is sativa-like, growing long, slender leaves and buds with abundant hairs. The frosty resin gives this plant a "sun dew" resemblance, with THC glands perched atop long stalks. Although usually a light to medium green, about 10 percent of the plants will exhibit some purple-blue coloration indicative of the Blueberry in the cross. This hybrid stays at a manageable height, usually ranging between 2-4 feet (60-120 cm).

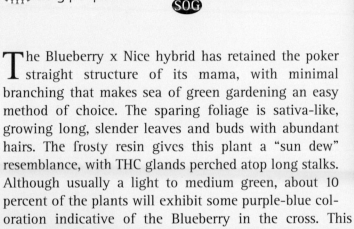

Blueberry x Nice has an intense, sweet-herbal aroma. The high is very potent but upbeat, making it great for conversation and long walks, or for unwinding after a long day. The yield is modest but quick—a satisfying addition to the indoor connoisseur's garden.

Most indoor methods are suitable for this plant, but Irish Rose prefers the use of an organic medium fertilized with an organic tea. Optimal conditions are a daytime temperature between 76-78 degrees F and a nighttime temperature of 56–65 degrees F with an overall humidity at 50 percent. Try vegetating plants at 18 hours of light, then flowering on an $11\frac{1}{2}$ hour light cycle to finish in 7 weeks.

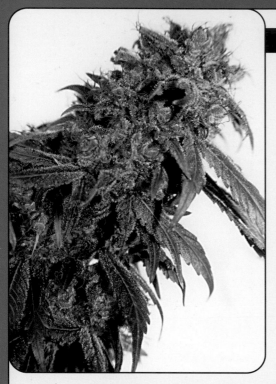

 56-63 days

 up to 125 g per plant in; up to 1lb per plant out

 Blueberry x Northern Lights

 cerebral

 berry

This hybrid is a backcross that consists of 75 percent Northern Lights from Holland and the U.S. Pacific Northwest, and 25 percent Blueberry from DJ Short's Delta 9 Collection. The result is a plant with a complex high and an appealing balance of physical and cerebral effects. Blueberry genetics have added the telltale berry aroma and occasional blue-purple tones to this otherwise Northern Lights–like plant.

Growth patterns generally resemble the indica-dominant Northern Lights, with a few exceptions. As with Northern Lights, this hybrid has a short stature with wide-fingered leaves and dense, pungently sweet flowers. The plant growth tends to elongate more than NL, which is the Blueberry's influence. These girls may also make more branches, which are thinner than the typically straight, thick main stem of Northern Lights.

As a result, Blueberry x Northern Lights is less suitable than many varieties for a sea of green method, giving more appreciable results as a larger indoor plant. Dr. Atomic favors staking multiple branched plants in 5-gallon pots of soil. This one will also thrive outdoors. Blueberry x Northern Lights is a strong, hardy plant, a good selection for the neophyte grower who wants an easy-to-maintain, larger plant offering a complex high with a strong cerebral effect and a berry aroma and flavor.

45-55 days in mid-Sep to early Oct out

22.5 g per f2 with 40 wpf in; 250 g per plant out

 Highland Thai (f) x Afghan Indica (m)

 giggly, munchies, sleepy

fruity/acrid

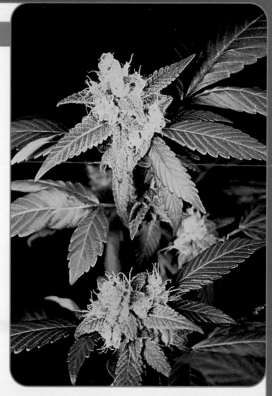

The name Blue Moonshine originated in a dream. The variety that inherited this dream-inspired moniker reveals mostly indica characteristics in structure and potency. Blue Moonshine is a short, stout, bushy plant. Outdoors, it rarely exceeds 3 feet (one meter), and is rarely over 2.5 feet (75 cm) indoors. One advantage of this variety is that it may be cropped quite low indoors or out.

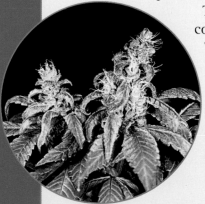

The leaves are dark and wide. This plant produces dense, sticky buds, coated with tall-standing, glandular stalked trichomes—a true "hash plant." The aroma and flavor of both the growing bud and the finished product is strong and astringent with a distinct fruity or fermented fruity taste.

In its effect, Blue Moonshine is akin to the homebrew that its name brings to mind. It is a potent smoke with a strong sensation of expansion in the lungs that is likely to induce coughing. The high is long lasting and physical, commonly beginning with hilarity, followed by extreme appetite stimulation then sedation.

Because genetics determine a plant's potential, selecting varieties is a major decision that should not be underestimated. Strains have multiple qualities for which they can be selected. Qualities that may influence selection include the type of high and the taste and smell, as well as growing characteristics and yield. While many varieties will perform acceptably in all of these categories, it is impossible to maximize each factor, so it is necessary to prioritize the importance of each before making a selection.

Today, most varieties available are fairly high in potency. Since that's the case, the quality of the high is often more important than sheer strength. In general, an indica or indica-dominant strain tends to have a somewhat sedating effect and a sativa has an "up" or "cerebral" type of high. Many strains of marijuana are indica/sativa hybrids that blend indica and sativa characteristics. For a variety that has a certain taste or smell, such as orange for example, the plant description should be helpful in narrowing the selection.

Growing characteristics and yield are important factors in their own right. A strain that is delicate and requires a lot of care may overwhelm the casual gardener. Pure sativas typically take a very long time to finish flowering. While indicas typically finish after 7 or 8 weeks of flowering, a pure sativa may take as long as 16 weeks. Some experts say this is because sativas are found in the tropics where the growing season is long.

Some strains are easier to clone than others. A plant that flowers at a certain age even under 24-hour light will not root readily when cloned. This characteristic, called auto-flowering, indicates a poor candidate for cloning. Again, the plant's description and the seed distributor should be able to provide information about this factor.

Seeds should be carefully examined. Good seeds are fairly dark in color and have dark

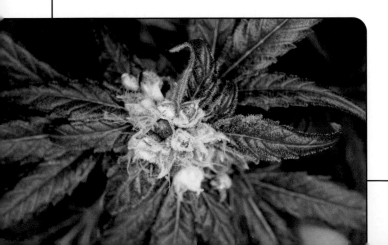

brown or black markings. These markings may be in the form of spots or stripes. This shows they are mature with a higher probability of sprouting. Poor seeds are pale, white or green without markings and have a low probability of germinating. Also to be avoided are seeds that are cracked or very small or shriveled in appearance. Seeds of the same type often have similar markings that vary from seed to seed. There is no way I know of to determine male from female by examining the seeds themselves. Likewise, sativa or indica can't be reliably determined by appearance. Good seeds sprout, or germinate, at the rate of 80–100 percent but there is no way to be sure which will sprout and which won't.

Some companies advertise what are called "feminized" seeds, which are said to produce all-female offspring. These do work but the results vary and one can't count on 100 percent female plants. Good seeds properly aged sprout 1–3 days after being placed in soil. Older seed may take up to 2 weeks to sprout. The best way to store seeds is to keep them in the refrigerator and keep them dry. Dried rice or silica gel can be used as a desiccant. Seeds stored this way keep for years, possibly decades, with only a slight reduction in germination rate.

Outside of marijuana-tolerant societies like Holland, initial selections have to be determined from the reputation and descriptions provided by companies, or other reliable sources. Therefore, the best approach is to try several varieties to determine the one or ones that are most satisfactory. Seed vendors in countries where seeds are sold legally often can be contacted via the Internet. Being well informed is key. Checking with a seedbank rating service can help one sidestep the dishonest companies out there. An honest and highly regarded seedbank will offer a quality product and top-notch customer service.

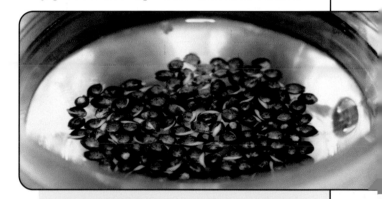

The author has been writing columns and rating seedbanks under the pseudonym **Green Man** since 1997. Green Man also provides grow advice on Usenet and message boards, and has been cultivating the green for over 20 years. His non-affiliated seedbank ratings offer a great service for the careful consumer, and can be accessed at www.seedbankupdate.com.

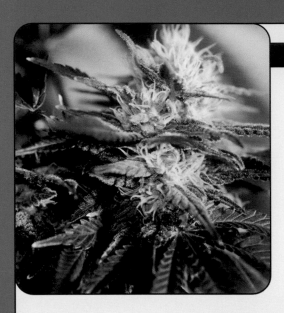

Blue Skunk Special

I S 80/20

53-58 days in
65-72 days out
or greenhouse

175-225 g per plant

Blueberry #1 x
Northern Lights #5

body relaxation

blueberry with
pepper

Blue Skunk Special was born when connoisseur breeder Krystal crossed Northern Lights #5 with a huge dominating male plant, the Blueberry #1, then backcrossed with Holland Skunk Special. Under optimum conditions this heavily indica hybrid is a big mama with large calyxes and purple-blue hues.

The "special" thing about Blue Skunk Special is that the skunk is in the name alone. The complex smell betrays no skunk heritage, instead giving off a berry aroma with a hint of spice and honeyed oil. Tasting of fruit and a dash of pepper, Blue Skunk Special's buzz is very kicked back and smooth, a deep couch potato stone. While this variety tends to keep a medium height, she has a stocky build with copious branching and large fan-shaped leaves.

Blue Skunk Special does especially well in an indoor professional environment or greenhouse. Once mistaken for an orange tree at first glance when growing in a greenhouse, the scent nevertheless makes it hard to miss her true identity. Hydroponic and soil set-ups are equally suitable. The tendency to branch makes it best suited as a large multiple branch plant, but Blue Skunk can be tamed to work in a sea of green method. This plant also fares well in the great outdoors, growing as tall as 6 feet (2 meters).

Blue Velvet

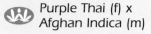 50/50

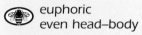 45-55 days in early-late Oct out at 45° N

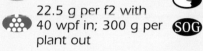 22.5 g per f2 with 40 wpf in; 300 g per plant out

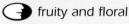 Purple Thai (f) x Afghan Indica (m)

euphoric even head–body

fruity and floral

SOG

Blue Velvet is a "leggy" half sativa–half indica cross, named for her lush appearance. Due to the lineage, this variety has also been known as Blueberry Thai. The long branches sport lavender-red leaves and the buds have a trademark "fox tail" appearance. The calyxes are large and striped.

Very enjoyable to the nose and palate, Blue Velvet's fragrance and flavor border between fruity and floral. Expect an uplifting and euphoric experience with this variety. The buzz gives both a head and body sensation, making it good for daytime use, socializing with friends, or for creative solitary ventures.

Because of its height and minimal foliage, Blue Velvet is recommended for a sea of green method. This variety will also grow lovely tall plants outdoors, reaching as high as 9 feet (3 meters) when supported and not cropped, or 6 feet (2 meters) wide when trellised. Outdoor plants can produce up to 300 grams of dried bud when the growing season is long enough to accommodate a mid-fall harvesting time.

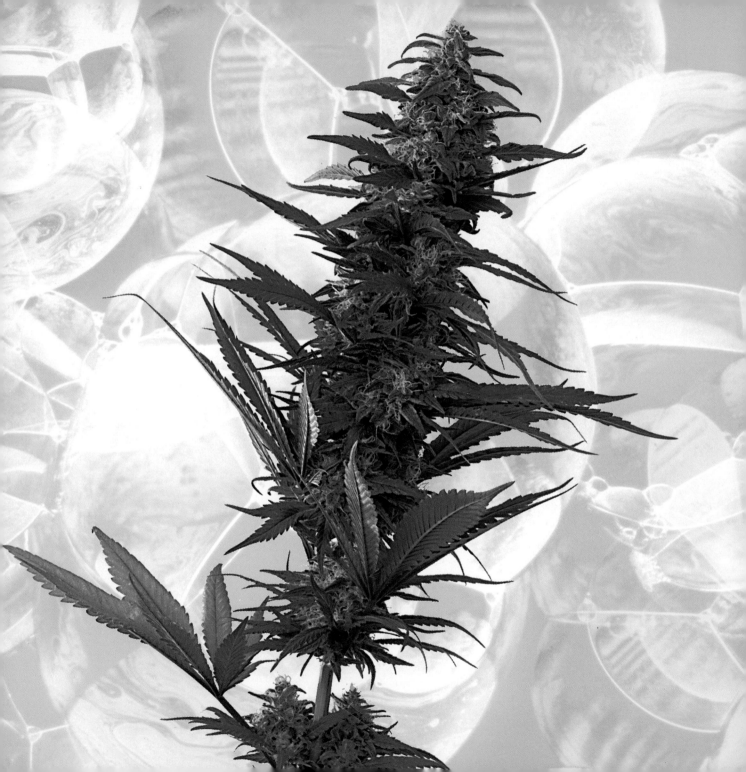

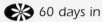

Bubbleberry

 80/20

 60 days in

 300-325 g per m2

Bubble Gum x Blueberry

euphoric and cheerful

pungent and skunky

SOG

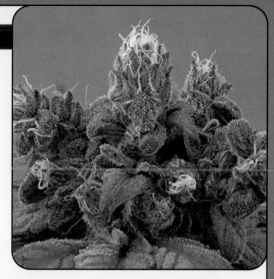

The name Bubbleberry is a merging of its parent variety names, Bubble Gum and Blueberry. Likewise, Bubbleberry has merged many of their favorable characteristics. The Bubbleberry variety owes its uniform growth pattern, large size, thick sturdy stem, and sticky resinous flowers to mother Bubble Gum, who came to Holland via Indiana and Rhode Island. Papa Blueberry passed along the down-to-the-calyx purple hues and the flavor that is made more complex by the Bubble Gum influence.

Bubbleberry's taste is rich and smooth with a hint of fruit. On and off the plant, the scent is skunky and pungent, making Bubbleberry less appropriate for covert public smoking or taking risks for outdoor growing with neighbors nearby. The Bubbleberry buzz is cheerful, and can be counted on to chase your funk away.

This strain is recommended for beginners as well as the experimental grower looking for a variety with dependable, generous results. A thick-stemmed, straight grower that resists spider mites with gusto, Bubbleberry is happy in many growing environments, including the sea of green method, which will provide beautiful single colas.

A flagship variety for the grower, Bubbleberry has been a longstanding favorite at Amsterdam's Grey Area coffeeshop, where it created lines around the block after receiving an honorable mention and intriguing write-up at the Cannabis Cup in the mid-1990s.

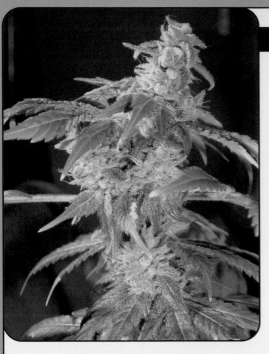

Bubble Gum

 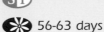 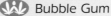 Bubble Gum

 56-63 days uplifting

  sweet

SOG: 450 g per m2 SOG

The Bubble Gum originated in Indiana in the 1970s. After making the rounds in the states, the genetics were taken to Holland during the 1990s, where a stable interbred variety was developed. Named Bubble Gum from the start, this variety quickly acquired a reputation for its sweetness, so much so that the name "Bubble Gum" has been widely borrowed for all sorts of seeds and weed.

There are two typical Bubble Gum plant structures: a pole plant with a main branch and minimal side branching, and a more natural evergreen shape with more branching from the main stem. Plants with almost no side branching should be forced to flower early and clipped to control height. Needless to say, these branchless beauties lend themselves perfectly to a sea of green system. Plants that exhibit branching are happy left with multiple branches. Although this means fewer plants per square meter and a longer maturation time, the plants will thank you with a higher yield.

A slow starter with less initial vigor than an f1 hybrid, Bubble Gum needs extra germination time. But don't veg for too long—she tends to stretch during flowering. Serious recommends indoor soil methods for a healthier harvest. Sporting beefy colas and stems strong enough to support them, Bubble Gum gains red hues at maturation. You may be surprised by how much the scent reminds you of genuine bubblegum.

The winner of many accolades, Bubble Gum has placed repeatedly in the *High Times* Cannabis Cup: 3rd place in 1994 for best coffeeshop product, 2nd place for best bioproduct and 2nd for the overall Cannabis Cup in 1995, and 2nd place again in 1999 for the overall Cannabis Cup.

Buddha's Sister

I

63-70 days

25-30 g per plant
in 1 gal. pot

Reclining Buddha x
Afghani Hawaiian

cerebral

tart fruity candy

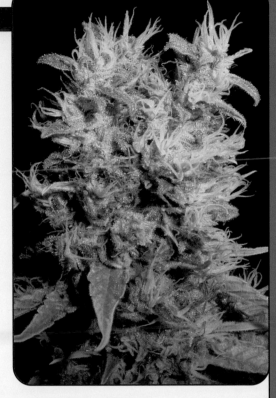

Previously called Soma Skunk V+, this variety was renamed Buddha's Sister to suit her tendencies and advance her appeal to Amsterdam coffeeshops. What's in a name? Directly after this deliciously good weed acquired a more intriguing name, she regularly sold out at the coffeeshops, and remains one of the best selling weeds available at De Dampkring.

This botanical sibling of Siddhartha is tall and lanky. In the cross with Afghani Hawaiian, she has gained considerably in yield, but has lost some of the sweetness of her other half, the Reclining Buddha. Buddha's Sister has a flavor like a tart cherry candy, and the scent is similarly tart. The buds have a slippery, silky feel, which means an abundance of greasy resin to transform into fantastic hash. She even gives a lot of finger hash that you won't want to wash away after grooming plants. As with all of Soma's varieties, Buddha's Sister is medicinal quality cannabis, therapeutic for many conditions. The high is powerful, creative and cerebral in its effects.

A mostly indica variety, Buddha's Sister tends to make lots of side branches, so she is better to grow as a multi-branch plant instead of in a sea of green. She will thrive using a sea of green method with some attentiveness. This variety does well hydroponically, but Soma's totally organic soil methods also deliver great results.

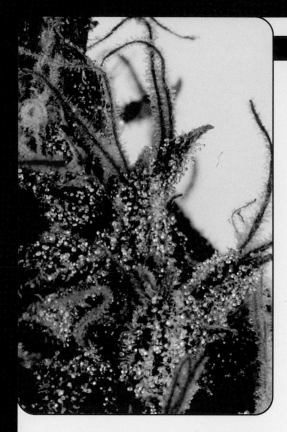

California Indica

 I

 45-50 days in early Oct out or greenhouse

450 g per m2 in
500 g per plant out

 Home and Hash Plant x Northern Lights #1 hybrid

 stoney

fruity/acrid

California Indica's mother was chosen from the original true-breeding Afghani lines from Sensi Seeds. After years of selective breeding, Home was selected as the mother. Home is very much like California Sweet Orange bud, but the flowers aren't as dense. By hybridizing with two heavy indica strains, the resulting California Indica produced sweet, pungent heavy buds with lots of resin.

California Indica has less foliage than most Sensi varieties, with a nice flower structure that is open and airy. The bud's hairs will turn orange upon drying. The buzz is a pleasant body relaxer with mellow effects that won't lock you on the couch after one toke. With a sweet yet pungent aroma and mostly sweet flavor, California Indica is the least "green" and the most "orange" strain that Sensi offers.

California Indica gives the best yields in the shortest time in a hydro culture garden. This plant can be grown in the sea of green style, but performs optimally when allowed to develop multiple branches. Remember that light and space are equally important in determining yield. Changes to these conditions change the yield by as much as 125 g per m2. While only appropriate for some outdoor climates, this strain has performed admirably in Spain and other dry Mediterranean type climates. Even indoors, you are best advised to keep your room a little on the dry side to avoid mold with this variety. Despite this, California Indica is a tolerant, versatile plant which performs well under many conditions.

80/20

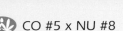 CO #5 x NU #8

 49-63 days

 uplifting

 sweet

 variable by grower

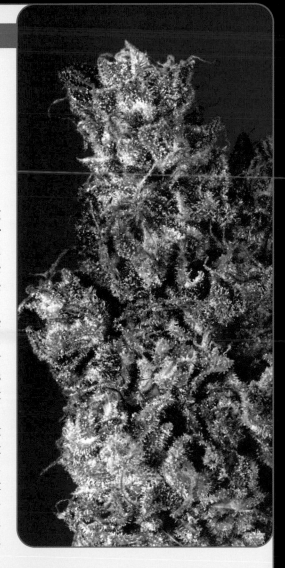

Caramella is a stable, mostly indica hybrid with long colas and a fresh caramel scent that accounts for her storybook name. Bred for the last 15 years with much success, she was selectively backcrossed for taste and a high calyx-to-leaf ratio. Caramella is a stable strain that gives homogeneous results.

Fresh, deep green leaves turn dark in color as she matures, making Caramella the picture perfect plant. The stems on this plant are thick and strong, easily supporting the big fat tops. You can also count on lots of dewy crystal formation scattered like faerie dust along the leaves and buds.

Caramella offers an uplifting and social high, great for a night out with friends. It smells like sweet caramel candy, which also comes through in the flavor. The smooth sweet taste may surprise you—for best results on optimizing the flavor, choose fertilizers carefully and use them modestly. Overfertilization encroaches on the flavor and the smoke is harsher on the lungs.

Caramella is robust and easy to grow, performing equally well in a hydro or soil system. This strain has the promising yield potential of a solid indica. Homegrown Fantaseeds advises 20 plants per square meter when using a sea of green method.

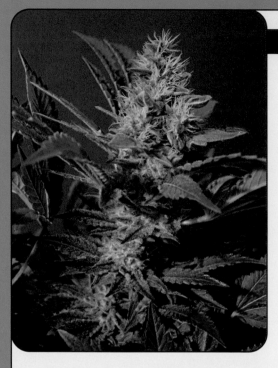

Chocolate Chunk

 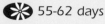

 55-62 days

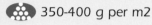

350-400 g per m2

 California selected indica

 narcotic, strong

 hashy chocolate

As the name suggests, Chocolate Chunk is a chunky, solid indica that has a deep hashy flavor with a touch of bittersweet chocolate and a narcotic bite. The plant has an electric green color that darkens to a deep green as it matures. Its super-wide leaves and exaggerated structure remove any doubt that it is a true indica.

While listed as a special-made indoor variety for Europe, this plant has outperformed other varieties when grown outdoors in the U.S. This is a great plant to cross with when creating hybrids, especially if you have something that's good but is either not producing enough or not dense enough.

With a finishing time of 8 weeks, Chocolate Chunk yields a very smooth smoking bud. The smell of the dried product is deep, but not too musky. This variety is low on the totem pole of smell—with proper ventilation and minimal disturbance to the plants, Chocolate Chunk can be relatively smell-free throughout the growing cycle. As with many pure indicas, she may tend to hold a lot of water so mind your watering to increase success.

4th place, *High Times* Cannabis Cup 2000

Adam from TH Seeds on the Hunt for Chocolate Chunk:

"I was looking for a chocolatey flavor. TH Seeds went out on a mission for that flavor, and it's the hardest flavor to find. California was the obvious choice for undertaking the search because we had the most contacts there. The variety we eventually chose originated in Oregon.

We wanted a chocolate flavor on the lighter side because indicas tend to have a very green flavor, no matter what you do, since the plant is such a high chlorophyll producer. If you take your typical indica, it's a very wide leaf, a heavy green, a dark, dark, dark color. You take your typical equatorial sativa, it's all light, so the flavors are much easier to bring out. We were looking for an indica that didn't have a very heavy sweet smell with a very heavy, not-so-sweet taste, which is what you often get with the indicas.

Chocolate Chunk is an Afghan cross—incidentally, the male is from the same family as the SAGE male, but not as extreme as the SAGE daddy. Since Chocolate Chunk was already hardy it wasn't necessary to find another heavy hitter for the cross. We were looking for something that gave some resin. The male we selected actually produces resin on the male to the naked eye, you can actually see some on the male. That's an achievement in and of itself because the males don't usually get to that point.

The growth pattern was also really important because most indicas can get very leafy to the point of no yield. You may have a room that's absolutely chock-full, but when you actually harvest . . . that's when it really pays to have something with a little more space between the buds, between the sites and the nodes. Sometimes people get this idea that all you need is a very close, tight plant to produce a lot of weight. In reality that's why some of the hybrids tend to work better—the spacing allows for a better harvest. Since this one is a pure indica we wanted to retain the strong indica characteristics as much as possible. We didn't want a real leggy plant, but we also didn't want to end up with something too similar to the Northern Lights type of plants that are fairly commonplace now. We wanted something unique."

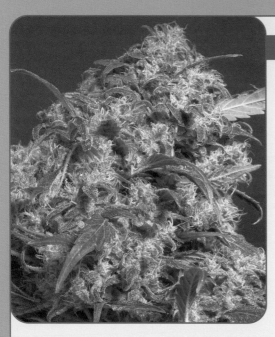

Chronic

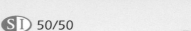

 50/50

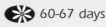 60-67 days

400-600 g per m2

SOG

 Northern Lights, Skunk x Northern Lights, AK-47

 even body–head

floral

Chronic is serious flower power. This easy-to-grow plant can produce up to 600 g per square meter under 600 watt lights; that's a gram per watt. These desirable yields have been achieved with both hydro and soil methods. Hydro methods require less time in vegetative stage, around 3 days, whereas fledglings need about a week to get rooted in soil. Chronic wants to grow a huge end bud, and any side buds are much smaller, making it a perfect candidate for the sea of green method. Chronic colas are impressively monstrous, getting as big as a typical forearm. Serious Seeds advises against clipping to promote bigger side buds, which will result in a decreased yield.

This once predominantly indica breed has been updated with a sativa cross and stabilizing since 2000, which improved both the strength and resin content, while leaving the subtle sweet-spicy scent intact. The high has a full spectrum of effects that typically start in the mind and then move to the body. This variety has a light wildflower scent and flavor with almost no trace of pungency or tang. The smell is subtle when the plant is alive and can be enhanced to a delicious sweetness if cured and dried properly.

Chronic has shown two phenotypes in the past. Plants have typically been either short with chubby buds or thinner with more elongated, slightly fluffed buds on taller plants. Since the breeding work at the start of the new century, Chronic has become more uniform, resembling the latter, more elongated type. The buds are also denser and more resinous than before. Chronic flowers early, and shows gender easily, with good sized preflowers at the base of the fan leaves along the stem. This variety won 3rd place in the 1994 *High Times* Cannabis Cup in the hydro division.

Simon on the Chronic:

"Along with AK-47 and the original Kali Mist, Chronic was bred in the days when Serious still had an enormous space to conduct experiments: the early 1990s. Chronic was first developed in 1994 with the goal of producing a plant that combined quality with a good yield. Up until that point, it seemed like there was some discrepancy between these two selection characteristics, and growers often had to sacrifice one for the other. I wanted to create a variety that proved this idea wrong, something that produced enormous buds without compromising a quality high for an enjoyable flavor or vice versa.

After its introduction, Chronic won 3rd place in the *High Times* Cannabis Cup in the hydro division—that was the only time it was entered in the Cup. But many other power-hitting indica strains have been released since 1994 that follow along the same lines, offering up both quality and yield with a mostly indica stone. By the late 1990s, Chronic seemed 'dated.' I decided it was time to give it a little more complexity and refresh this variety without losing any of the characteristics that made it so well-liked to start out with. I bred more sativa into the indica-dominant Chronic, which gave it a more complex, full-spectrum high without losing the nice yield and flavor. The facelift also improved both the strength and resin content.

The mildly sweet scent with a bit of spiciness also stayed intact, but curing and drying are fundamental to carrying this characteristic from the live plant to the smokeable product. Even while living, the wild-flower scent is subtle, but it will be lost for good if not dried properly. When put in plastic before completely dry, the scent is irreversibly gone, more so for this variety than for any others I've worked with. But if you let it dry thoroughly, the aroma develops a very strong, sweet smell which doesn't fade. This could be the difference between thinking Chronic is okay or fabulous pot for flavor connoisseurs."

Critical Mass

 S I

 45-55 days in mid-Sep out

 650-750 g per m2

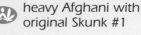 heavy Afghani with original Skunk #1

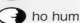 strong

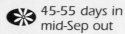 ho hum

Named for its heavy production, this plant literally produces the critical mass yield—the most you could hope to get before the plant's own branches snap from an inability to support its growth.

Critical Mass is a remastering of Big Bud for Mr. Nice Seed Bank. It has a genetic pedigree originating from a particularly heavy Afghani combined with the original Skunk #1. This is a seriously indica-like plant with thick-shaped leaves. In height and structure, it is medium-sized with a very high flower-to-leaf ratio.

Critical Mass gives a massive yield with an equally high stone. With a little luck, the experienced grower should be able to yield up to 750 grams per square meter indoors. Due to its heavy flower construction, it can be susceptible to mold in humid growing conditions. This risk is reduced by paying attention to humidity in indoor grows, and harvesting on time indoors or out.

While Critical Mass is low on resin production and lacks an especially distinctive taste, you'll be impressed with this heavy producer whose colas border on the obscene in their size and heft.

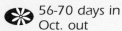

 I

 56-70 days in Oct. out

 out preferred

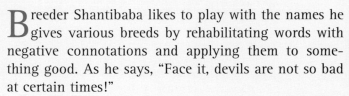 450-550 g per m2

 Afghan x Afghan/ Skunk cross

 psychedelic and uplifting

 fruity (apple) smell/ skunky taste

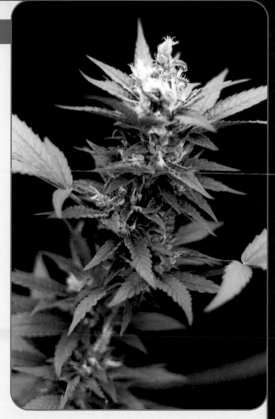

Breeder Shantibaba likes to play with the names he gives various breeds by rehabilitating words with negative connotations and applying them to something good. As he says, "Face it, devils are not so bad at certain times!"

This Devil's Afghani pedigree has given it a reddish aura that deepens as it matures. The leaves turn purple to red, like the colors of autumn, and are typically thick and fan-like in shape. The bud is a cluster of flowers and goes from dark green to purple to red as it finishes. Unlike many Afghani's, this hybrid is only a moderate resin producer.

The buzz will take you on a magical mind journey that can be wonderfully therapeutic and uplifting. This Devil is a good companion for exciting and adventurous undertakings. The bouquet is sweet like an apple orchard, while the taste also includes the parental skunk influence.

An easy-to-grow plant, Devil is recommended for the novice and is a great selection for outdoor or greenhouse growers. Although it shows slow growth initially, watch out once it has established its root ball. This plant finishes by October in the Northern hemisphere, June/July in the Southern hemisphere. If you try this one indoors, it must be placed in vegetative growth for at least 2 weeks if yield is the prime directive.

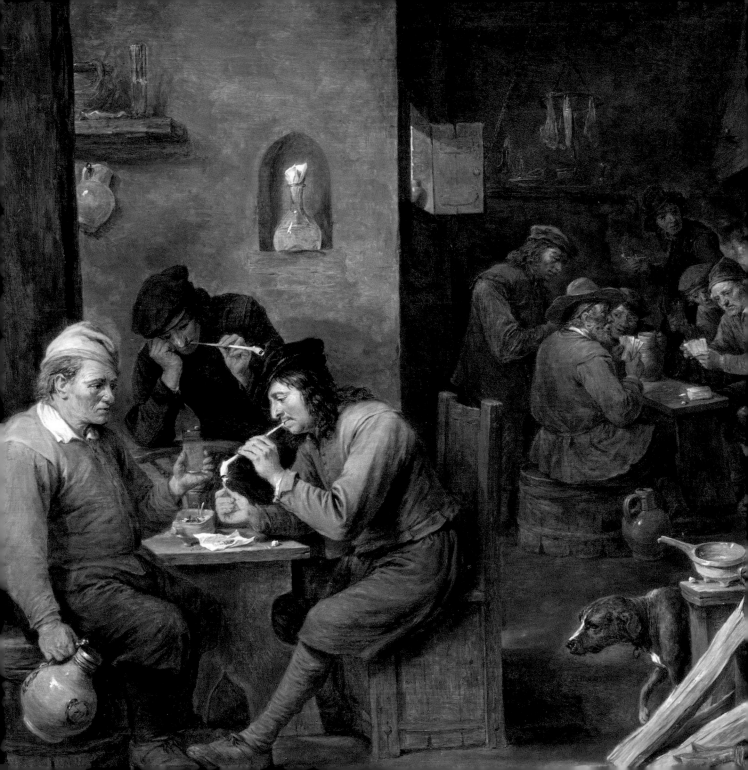

A History of Cannabis in Holland

Ben Dronkers with special thanks to Anne Bonney

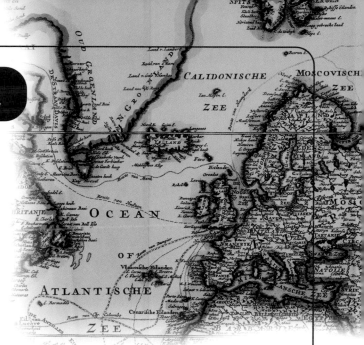

The breeding and selling of marijuana and cannabis seeds occurs in many places around the globe, but the Netherlands, and Amsterdam in particular, remains the epicenter of the cannabis earthquake currently shaking up the planet. What unique set of influences allowed the Netherlands to become so prominent in the cannabis world?

There is evidence that the cannabis plant has been used in the Netherlands for hundreds, possibly thousands, of years. Early residents of the marshy areas that became the Netherlands had access to hemp plants for food, fuel and fiber. As the Dutch language evolved into its present form, one word came to describe any and all sorts of cannabis plants: *hennep*.

Dutch farmers began stretching their expensive imported tobacco with the leaves and flowers of the hennep plant in the early 1500s. At this time, we have no way of knowing how much THC was in those early plants, but there is a good chance that they contained some.

Hemp smoking peasants in a "Smoking House" (1660), by David Teniers de Jonge

The Netherlands has long been a haven for those whose political, religious or social values were not tolerated in other places. For generations, the Dutch culture has embraced the value of allowing others to live as they choose, so long as it doesn't interfere with the whole of society. Along with the political and social unrest of the 1960s came a (Western) worldwide explosion in the use of cannabis and psychedelics. Part of this cultural upheaval was due to travel. Many young Europeans left the comforts of home or university to travel to the exotic East. In those days, the world political situation was such that one could drive (or in some cases, hitchhike) from Europe to Tangiers, Delhi or Kabul, and many did. On their travels, the young adventurers adopted many foreign practices— from meditation to vegetarianism to hashish smoking. Soon hashish began to find its way back to Western Europe, with Amsterdam, Frankfurt and other cities becoming consumption and distribution centers.

Not surprisingly, the Dutch official reaction to this trend was rational and practical. By the mid-1970s, there was widespread use of marijuana, speed, heroin, LSD and other recreational drugs presenting various degrees of health risks to Dutch citizens. The then-Minister of Health and Interior, Irene Vorink, examined the medical and social studies of the harm caused by the various substances. Vorink noted that young people often experiment with tobacco, sex, alcohol and other drugs as a natural part of the maturation process. She wanted to reduce any potential harm, and she felt that Dutch youth faced the most danger. She decreed that cannabis was considerably less harmful than the other drugs and that the most common way to be introduced to drugs "harder" than cannabis was directly through the hard drug suppliers themselves. Vorink recommended that authorities stop prosecuting people for the consumption and sales of personal amounts of cannabis. She also took advantage of existing youth centers as places to permit the sales of small amounts of hashish and marijuana. It was in these youth clubs that the commercial coffeeshops of today were born.

Long before it became socially current or politically contentious, cannabis had certainly grown in the Netherlands, so it was logical that the smokers of the 1960s would try to grow

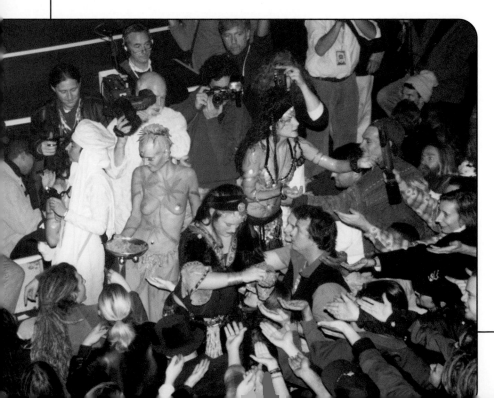

Cannabis Cup 1995
photo credit: Ed Rosenthal

their own. In the mid-1960s, artists Kees Hoekert and Jasper Grootveld fought the first symbolic battles to be permitted to grow cannabis. Their plants were leafy and low in potency, more rope than dope. By 1970, the Holland Hemp Company/Hookah Tribe was growing for buds. Even though seeds came from Thailand and Afghanistan, it was difficult to get anything very potent, largely because it is very hard to get mature buds outdoors in Holland before the autumn rain and cold kill the plants.

In 1978, people brought the first killer bud to the Netherlands from the States and a standard was established. The first good seeds from the States came in about 1980. The 1980s also saw the formation of Lowlands Seed Company, the Seed Bank, SSSC and Sensi Seeds. It was through the journalistic efforts of Ed Rosenthal that breeders started to communicate with each other, exchanging information and genetics. In 1985, strains developed in the U.S.—Skunk #1, Early Pearl, Original Haze, Northern Lights and Holland's Hope—were first grown in Dutch greenhouses. This revolutionized the growing and smoking scene.

Slowly but surely, as the potency increased, bud smoking began its rise in popularity in the Netherlands. In the mid-1980s Sensi

Seeds introduced large-scale cloning. By the end of the decade, the emphasis had shifted to production of green bud, from clones rather than seeds, to sell in coffeeshops or keep as personal stash. Imported hashish maintained its popularity throughout the 1980s, but sales of Dutch grown grass began

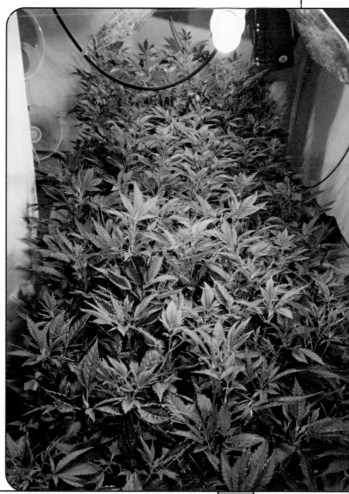

photo credit: Ed Rosenthal

to increase dramatically every year after 1985. By the early 1990s grass sales exceeded hash sales in most coffeeshops and continued to grow in share of the market until the mid-1990s. Shop owners have reported that since about 1996, they sell two grams of bud for every one gram of hashish sold. A small but growing number of Dutch smokers are adopting the North American practice of smoking their cannabis pure rather than the traditional hash and tobacco mix of Europe. As breeding advances and greater emphasis is placed on taste rather than potency, more smokers here may well "go pure."

The Dutch law made it possible to breed and produce seeds, but without the existing greenhouse industry and other farming techniques, the cannabis growers would not have moved ahead so fast. With the obstacles presented by Holland's weather addressed, the social and political climate made it a logical place for the industry to flourish. By the late 1980s, there was a quiet trade in seeds to the world from three or four busy companies. In 1987, U.S. smoker's magazine, *High Times*, started hosting a "Cannabis Cup." The event was modeled on the harvest festivals of the late 1970s and early 1980s in Northern California. A group of *High Times* writers evaluated the entries from various seed breeders and growers in Holland. In 1989,

the biggest trader was compromised by their U.S. contact and decided to shut down. The scene altered radically for a few years, with some major shifts of control over certain basic breeding strains. In the years following this breach, there wasn't much competition, so the Cup emphasis switched to the coffeeshops. The seed company competition was reinstated in 1994, with three firms entering varieties. By 2000, the number had risen to more than a dozen. At present, there is a multi-million-guilder cannabis seed industry in the Netherlands. Cannabis seeds have become just like tulips, vegetables, cheese and tomatoes—a major export product. In spite of the drug war, Holland still bombards the world with seeds.

Ben Dronkers is the founder and president of Sensi Seed Bank. He has been in the CannaBusiness since the early 1980s. His other endeavors include HempFlax, an industrial hemp firm and the Hash, Marijuana and Hemp Museum.

Anne Bonney is the namesake of the 17th century's most famous female pirate. She continues to subvert the dominant paradigm by writing intelligently about cannabis and other subjects.

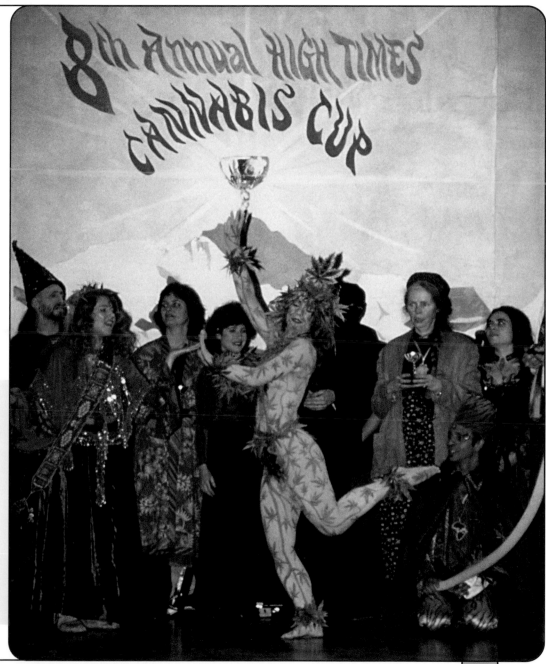

photo credit: Ed Rosenthal

Durga Mata

  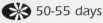

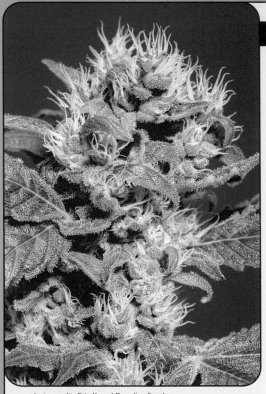

photo credit: Eric K and Paradise Seeds

I

 50-55 days

400-450 g per m2

SOG

 Cross of 2 Super Shivas

mellow

acrid, smelly, spicy

Named for the powerful and revered Hindu Mother Goddess, Durga Mata represents the purity and strength of purpose residing within the divine essence of every being. In Hindu tales, Durga Mata carries the sword of truth, destroying demons, conquering ignorance and leading humans to enlightenment.

The Paradise variety of Durga Mata will bring out your inner philosopher. The aroma is herbal and spicy, with a taste like Turkish fruit. The buzz is potent and physically relaxing, but will not necessarily put you to sleep. She is the quintessential after-dinner smoke for an evening of deep conversation with friends.

Durga Mata's Shiva parents were selected for their high resin content and ease in growth and maintenance. The variety is reliably homogeneous, with clone-like results that make it perfect for a sea of green set-up. These plants don't stretch much upon flowering. If grown vegetatively for 2 weeks, they may shoot up another foot while flowering. The internode spacing is tight and the buds are dense, compact, and grow very uniformly.

Durga Mata is not too finicky about her environment. Indoor growing on hydro, coco or soil is all good. She survives rough treatment and still performs very well, making this variety an excellent choice for newbies or medical growers. Durga Mata is recommended outdoors in temperate latitudes with mild climates, but has been grown in Holland with fine results.

Dutch Dragon

 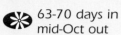 75/25

 63-70 days in mid-Oct out

 Skunk/Durban (f) x California indica (m)

 even body-head

 fruity/sweet

500 g per m2 in 600-700 g per plant out

SOG

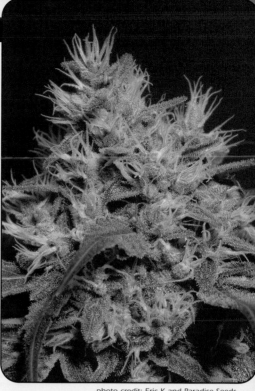

photo credit: Eric K and Paradise Seeds

Bred by Paradise Seeds in 1994, Dutch Dragon was developed in East Holland by crossing a stabilized Skunk/Durban hybrid female with a California indica father. A tall plant of fine sativa quality, Dutch Dragon has superb yields from long sticky colas. The aroma is very fruity and sweet, as is the taste. The buzz is a lasting high that increases one's appetite for music and pleasure.

Dutch Dragon performs best in warm climates growing into a tall plant with smallish fan-shaped leaves. A sea of green flowering cycle can be started early because Dutch Dragon is a quick growing plant with a typical sativa growth pattern. If height is a concern in your grow room, flower-forcing early is the best solution. For best results the pH should always be kept below 6.

Though fast out the gate, Dutch will take 9–10 weeks to develop big, fully matured flowers. When grown outside mid-October is favorable for harvesting this dragon, who can get as tall as 9 feet (3 meters). She can stretch to reach a height of almost 3 feet (80-90 cm) if grown using the sea of green technique.

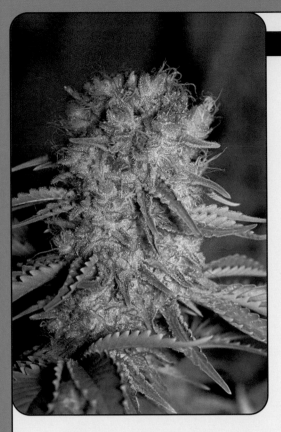

Dutchmen's Royal Orange

 I

 63-77 days in Oct out

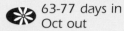

 up to 500 g per m2

 Skunk #1 (m) x California Orange (f)

 body relaxation, clear head

very sweet citrus

Dutchmen's Royal Orange has an international heritage. The Skunk #1 father was a stable hybrid of a Mexican/Colombian mother bred with a pure Afghan strain father. Royal Orange's indica mother, California Orange, originally came from Afghanistan by way of California. These parents were brought together by a legendary breeder in Holland in 1985.

This regal variety has a delectably sweet smell combined with a hashish taste exposing the Afghani mother's influence. The Royal Orange buzz is a strongly physical sensation good for kicking back in the sun, or on the couch for a long epic movie. Even with the strong bodily sensation, this variety retains the clear high of the Skunk parent.

Dutchmen's Royal Orange leaves are shiny and dark, with a typical indica plant structure overall—relatively short and wide with broad leaves. The buds are tight rocky nuggets, which along with the minimal vegetation makes this a high yielder. Despite this density, Royal Orange has terrific mold resistance and is very uniform in its growth habits, making it ideal for greenhouse cultivation. Flying Dutchmen recommends growing in soil using organic methods for best results.

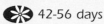

Early Queen

 42-56 days

 600-650 g per m2

SOG

Early Pearl x
Early Girl x
Super Skunk

giggly, eyedroop

minimal

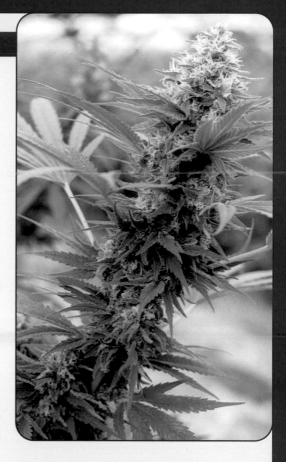

Since the beginning of the 1990s, this three-way hybrid has earned acclaim in the cultivators' world. Early Queen's genetic composition stems from a cross between early Californian blends mixed with African and a touch of Mexican. As an indica, Early Queen's leaves are fat and fan-like, and her straight, bushy stature usually grows to a medium height.

This strain's buds are large and crystally at the end, with yellow hairs. Early Queen focuses her energy on one main, large cola that forms quicker than many varieties because of its Durban line influence. The buzz is giggly and can make everything suddenly seem funny, but also may leave you feeling heavy in the eyelids.

True to the promise of her name, Early Queen is quick to finish both indoors and out, and is therefore an excellent selection for cold climate countries in the Northern hemisphere where she can finish as early as September (Southern hemisphere finish in March). Because of her speedy finish, she is a favorite among commercial growers. She also handles humidity well, making it possible for those in the world's wetter regions to produce a good outdoor product. In hot dry climates, growers will be gratified by the capacious harvest in a short time.

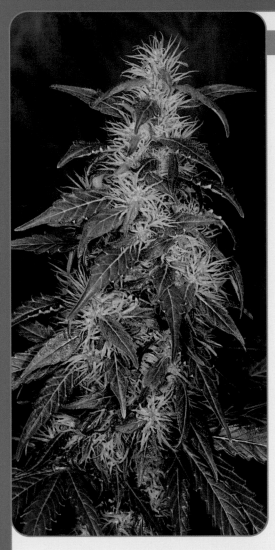

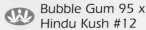

 60/40

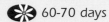 60-70 days

 varies

SOG

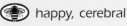 Bubble Gum 95 x Hindu Kush #12

 happy, cerebral

 fruity!

E clipse is a new variety from Homegrown, a mostly sativa hybrid with a sweet taste and long tendrils of hair on the buds. It has commonalities with the notorious Bubble Gum.

A great variety for the young or young at heart, Eclipse offers clear, jubilant effects. The buzz creates a mind expanding sensation, which makes it great for meditation or other activities that would benefit from an enhanced sense of concentration. It has one of the fruitiest tastes that can be achieved and smells unbelievably fruity when growing.

This plant's height is easily controlled. Yield is dependent on growing skill, but Eclipse can harvest generously for a dominantly sativa hybrid. A great home grower variety, Eclipse does well in hydroponic or soil systems. Don't be tempted to harvest before these girls have reached full maturity. Eclipse needs a full 8½ weeks before she's ready, but has a safety zone for guerilla gardeners. This variety will stand as long as 10 weeks without any problems, if harvesting should be delayed. Leaving Eclipse for a full 10 weeks does not seem to improve the yield, taste, or offer any other notable advantage than the recommended 60 day harvest, but could come in handy if a long window of opportunity is needed. Eclipse's resin production, which is considerable, reaches its peak in the 8th week.

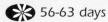

El Niño

 I S 60/40

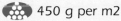 56-63 days

 Haze x Super Skunk Brazilian x South Indian

 sleepy

 citrus

450 g per m2

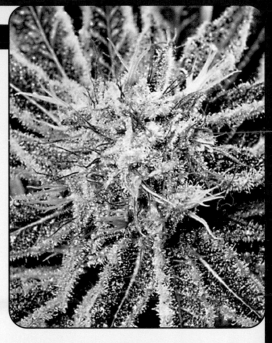

Developed by Greenhouse in 1996, El Niño is an indica/sativa hybrid of South American and Indian strains. This strain was stabilized and made available in 1998, the same year that it took first place at the *High Times* Cannabis Cup in the bioplant category.

Like the powerful weather phenomenon for which it was named, Greenhouse's El Niño washes over those who smoke it, creating a nearly overwhelming stoney sensation. A pacific variety, El Niño promises to alter your immediate atmosphere with a warm sociable feeling, but may also cloud your thinking with its sedating buzz. This strain is recommended as a tranquil nightcap to complete an evening.

El Niño is a medium to tall plant, with multiple branching and many budding sites. The short, fat flowers are resinous and have a strong lemon taste. Better as a multi-branch plant in an indoor garden, El Niño has a moderate yield potential. This crystally plant will also process well into hashish or kief.

The mostly equatorial origins of this plant make it suitable as an outdoor plant only within 40 degrees of latitude from the equator. Greenhouse recommends using hydroponic methods indoors for more temperate regions.

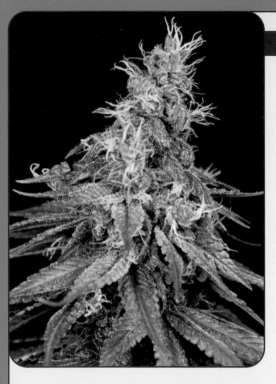

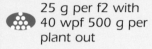

S I 60/40

42-49 days in end Sep out at 45° N

25 g per f2 with 40 wpf 500 g per plant out

  Purple Thai (f) x Afghan Indica (m)

active, cerebral

floral

A member of DJ Short's Delta 9 Blue Collection, Flo is an exciting plant. A sativa look-alike that matures early, Flo's name may reflect this plant's unique ability to produce a continual flow of buds through multiple harvesting.

Flo's large, tight, spear-shaped buds are made up of small, densely-packed, purple-striped calyxes. A very productive, fast maturing plant, Flo gets tall, and likes to branch out. The first buds are ripe by the end of September at or near the 45 parallel North. About every 10 to 12 days after reaching initial maturity, new buds form and can be harvested through the end of November, or as long as the plant can remain alive in the given outdoor conditions. Indoors, buds mature by the end of the 6th week of 12/12 light and are still producing mature buds into the 7th week. If you harvest only once, the yield will be more modest. Due to the Flo's multi-harvest potential, it is ideal for greenhouse production.

Flo has an energetic, motivating buzz with unusual clarity. This is true wake and bake pot, great to start the day off right without losing sight of your intentions. The flavor has a floral quality similar to Nepalese Temple Hash, with a touch of the blueberry tones that remind you they are relatives. The smell echoes the taste, remaining subtle and light. Flo was rated #1 at the 1996 Cannabis Cup by *Cannabis Culture* magazine.

The breeding and production of fine cannabis is more art than science. A creative mind and sense of intuition are necessary to achieve success in this field. While some herb is strictly pleasing to the mental palate, taste can also be tantamount to the buzz for the cannabis connoisseur.

The range of flavors expressed by the genus cannabis is extraordinary. No other plant on the planet can equal the cacophony of smells and tastes available from cannabis. The spectrum of possible smells and tastes a human can experience is large and complex. To date, no one has created a fully usable olfaction chart, although Ann Noble of the wine world has developed a nifty "aroma wheel" for that industry, which inspired me to develop a similar map for cannabis. Like its counterpart, categories branch out from the general to the more specific. For instance, a category like "fruity" will subdivide into "berry" and "citrus;" citrus divides further into the more distinct flavors of "lemon," "lime" and "orange."

The range of aromas and flavors represented on the chart (next page) are all possible to achieve. Some of these are already well known and represented among widely available cannabis varieties, while others require some cross-breeding to achieve. Some of the most desirable bud bridges multiple categories, creating a complex sensory experience. Although the strength of smell and flavor may vary, many strains' flavors were best expressed when they were grown outdoors in their region of origin. Note that aroma and flavor vary by growing method and also between various stages of the plant. The aroma of a live bud on the plant, a dried and cured bud, and the smoke on the inhale and exhale, may all be different from each other.

The physical palate of cannabis is a wondrous dimension, important in distinguishing the good from the superb in the weed world. Capable of being refined, one's palate is best educated through experience. The map that follows is meant to aid the discriminating stoner in charting the territory.

Happy travels.

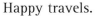

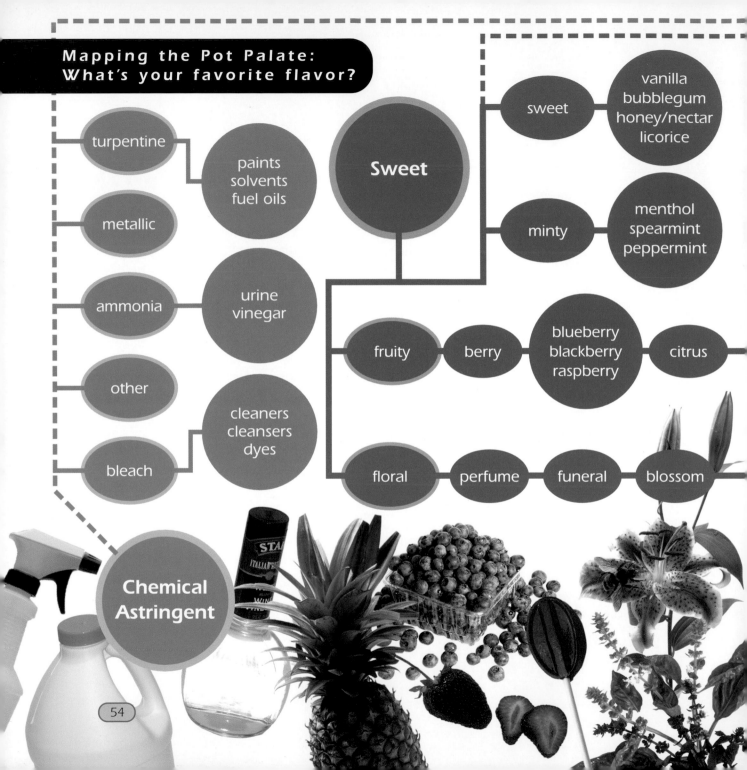

**Mapping the Pot Palate:
What's your favorite flavor?**

turpentine

metallic

paints
solvents
fuel oils

Sweet

sweet

vanilla
bubblegum
honey/nectar
licorice

minty

menthol
spearmint
peppermint

ammonia

urine
vinegar

fruity

berry

blueberry
blackberry
raspberry

citrus

other

cleaners
cleansers
dyes

bleach

floral

perfume

funeral

blossom

Chemical
Astringent

54

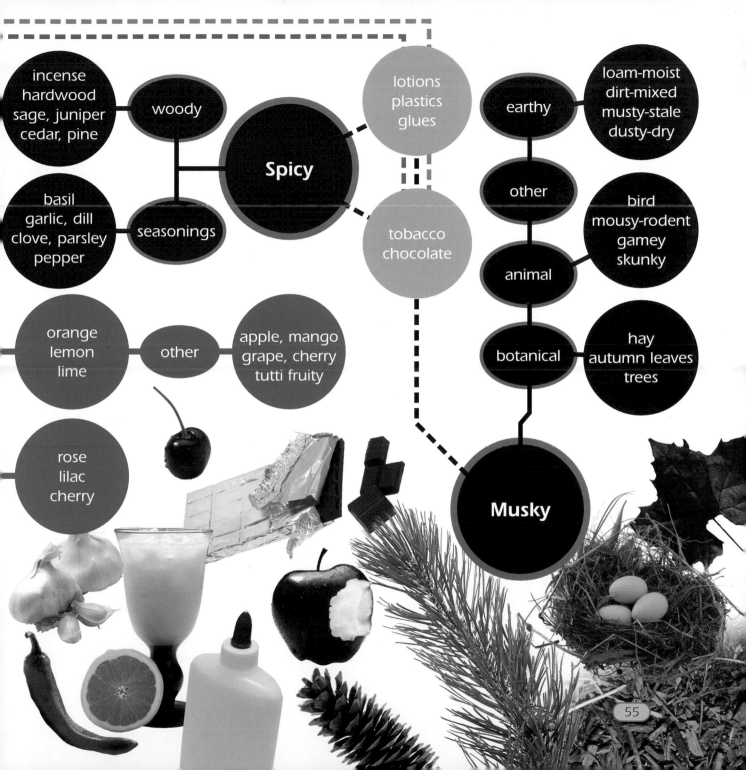

incense
hardwood
sage, juniper
cedar, pine

woody

lotions
plastics
glues

earthy

loam-moist
dirt-mixed
musty-stale
dusty-dry

Spicy

other

basil
garlic, dill
clove, parsley
pepper

seasonings

bird
mousy-rodent
gamey
skunky

tobacco
chocolate

animal

orange
lemon
lime

other

apple, mango
grape, cherry
tutti fruity

botanical

hay
autumn leaves
trees

rose
lilac
cherry

Musky

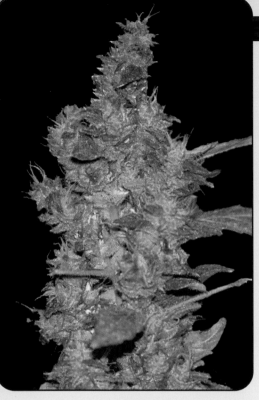

Hashmaster

 60/40

 70 days from rooted clone, 60 days soil in; Oct out

 SOG: up to 36 g per plant in; 120 g per plant out

 Hashmaster back crossed strain

 cerebral, munchies

skunky, earthy

SOG

Shaped like a classic Mexican pine, Hashmaster is a 60/40 sativa/indica hybrid revived through the backcrossing work of Doc Bush. This variety was originally purchased from Marc Emery in the mid-1990s, but became unavailable shortly afterward. After five backcrosses, Doc Bush's Hashmaster is now fully stabilized so that cross-pollinating seedlings will produce true Hashmaster seeds, avoiding wild f2 hybrids.

The branches of this strain can reach up to a foot indoors and as long as 4 feet outdoors. Hashmaster's leaves are large distinct fans with many dark green leaflets. Due to the massive size and easily identifiable skunk aroma that travels on the wind, outdoor guerilla growers should select their garden plot with care. The record outdoor yield for this strain was 3.6 pounds on one plant in the semi-tropics.

Hashmaster is a smooth and creamy smoke with a strong hash-like smell reminiscent of 1970s Afghani "Red Seal" pressed hash. This ganja is an earthy classic with a one-toke, cerebral, munchie-producing high. For hashish fans, the name alone should have you guessing that a little effort can result in some master hash.

Minimal vegetative growth is required to produce great results with Hashmaster. Indoor clones are flowered at 2-3 weeks. Doc Bush highly recommends trimming the lower branches for size control indoors. This strain's tendency to produce one large dominant cola make it a workable plant in a sea of green growing method when trimmed attentively.

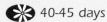

Hash Plant

 I

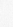 40-45 days

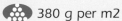

 380 g per m2

SOG

 Original Hash Plant x
Hash Plant/Northern
Lights #1 hybrid

 body stone

sweet/spicy

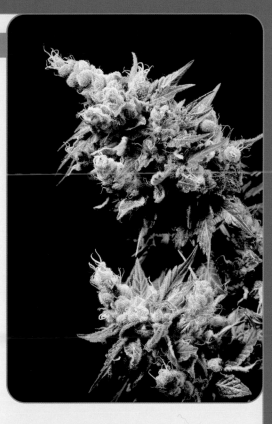

H ash Plant derives from the famed indoor Hash Plant cutting that traveled to Holland from the Northwest U.S in the 1980s. This hybrid was crossed to one of the three genotypes of the super Afghanis, Northern Lights #1, to produce an impressively strong indica specimen.

Named for its hashy-tasting, highly resinous buds, the Hash Plant has been known as an important building block for other Sensi Seeds hybrids for many years, but has rarely been made available outside of the Cannabis Castle breeding program. It was reintroduced to the market by the Sensi Seed Bank in 1999.

Expect a short indica-type plant that averages 3-4 feet (100-130 cm) in height, with a gratifyingly quick finish, a pleasantly narcotic high, and of course, great hashmaking potential.

While an indoor breed in the Dutch climate, this plant has fared well in dry latitudes such as the Mediterranean. All indoor growing methods are suitable, although Sensi growers like the hydro culture garden method best. Hash Plant is easy to clone, offering you a simple method for multiplying your success.

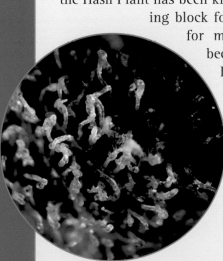

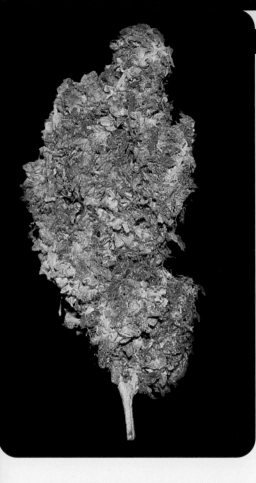

Hawaiian Haze

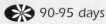

90-95 days

medium

Hawaiian x
secret indica

cerebral

floral

Hawaiian Haze's name tells its story of origins. This combination of a renowned Hawaiian island sativa with a Haze/indica hybrid has produced a pleasing tropical smoke with the smell of freshly cut flowers.

Although Hawaiian Haze contains some indica, the growth time, the high and the plant's structure all show strong sativa characteristics. The light tones of this plant are further paled by the clinging resin. Aroma and taste are similar to the Southeast Asian Haze variety, although they remain only softly floral. The leaves are elegant and thin, and the buds are small and airy. The high is also airy and cerebral, inspiring a euphoric mood and positively affecting the clarity of your thoughts.

Hawaiian Haze has inherited the tall stature typical of the Haze varieties. From the outset, seedlings should be grown under a 12/12 regimen of light to control the height in an indoor garden. With a 13-week-plus flowering time, this plant should not be attempted outside without the benefit of a long equatorial growing season. Hawaiian Haze's yield, while satisfying, is not likely to be your largest yielder, making this a more appropriate plant for the connoisseur gardener rather than the commercial grower.

Hawaiian Sativa

 S

  sativa

84 days

alert, cerebral

citrus

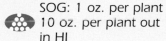 SOG: 1 oz. per plant
10 oz. per plant out
in HI

SOG

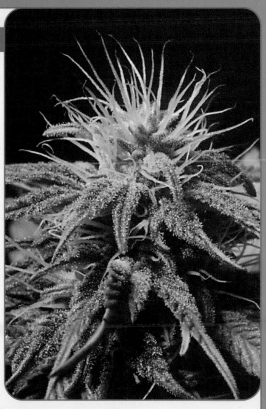

Hawaiian Sativa has the instincts of a canopy dweller, competing to outgrow surrounding vegetation. Fully stabilized after nearly 30 years of breeding, this variety has been described as "Banana Hawaiian pot" because of her thick, curved buds. Buds have very wispy sativa-like hairs, and elongated calyxes, giving this plant more than the usual number of trichomes per square centimeter. In other words, resin galore.

Limey green in color, Hawaiian Sativa is a poker-straight plant with minimal side branches. Good in a sea of green method when the height is controlled, this sativa will also thrive staked to poles, and can be planted densely in a small space using this method. If staking, tie a string around the outside to hold the plants together for best results.

Hawaiian Sativa's citrus flavor and menthol tingle will go to your head. For a more intense citrus flavor, hydroponics growers might try flushing with water for 3 weeks prior to harvest.

Because the high leaves your brain wide-awake and functional, she's a good candidate for those who can freely toke all day. Hawaiian Sativa possesses analgesic properties that have increased its popularity among medical patients seeking pain relief. Anecdotal evidence suggests that Hawaiian Sativa provides good visual ocular release, making it a preferred variety for glaucoma patients.

All these superlatives come at a price for the outdoor grower, as Hawaiian Sativa takes a good 84 days to mature and should not be harvested until early November outdoors unless you're in a rainy climate. Yields outside of the tropics are diminished in an outdoor grow.

Federation's Story about the Hawaiian Sativa:

"This variety came to me as a sativa, and was indigenous on Hawaii since the 1970s. It didn't make it over here to North America until the 1980s, because commercial growers are generally not interested with the more time-consuming sativa varieties. A lot of commercial growers want to grow indicas because it's quick, and they want the biggest bang for the buck. They just want to get the product out there in a shorter amount of time than a sativa allows for.

In the 1980s, a buddy of mine went over to Hawaii on his honeymoon, and met a giant Samoan guy on the beach. My buddy was sitting on the beach, smoking his little joint and the Samoan guy sniffs and says, 'Hey that smells all right. Let me have some of that.' My friend hands him the joint. He takes a puff, gives it back and says, 'Hmmph, that's nothin.'

The guy pulls out this great big huge gagger of a joint. They sit there smoking it together, and get totally wrecked. My friend comments that it was really kind stuff. The Samoan guy takes him back to his place, and in his back garden behind the house, he had these giant sativa plants. He broke my friend off some buds for later. When my buddy got back to his hotel room, he found that the bud was seeded, so he brought the seeds home and gave them to me. I grew them out, and once I knew it would give stable results, I made them available."

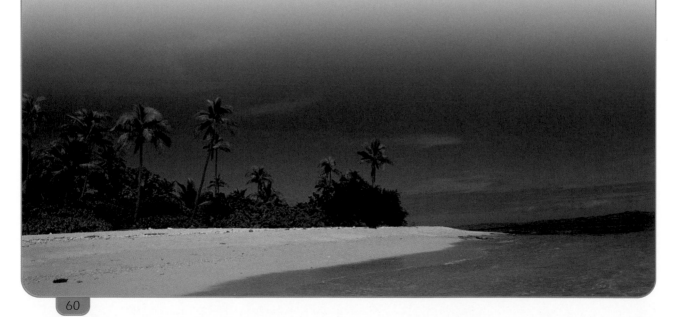

The Story Behind the Haze

In the 1970s, there were two brothers growing pot in Monterey, California who were known as the Haze Brothers. They were working on a super all-sativa strain that would do well in their location. They experimented, taking a variety of pure sativas and crossing them. A combination of several sativas, including a Mexican/Colombian and some Thai, resulted in a long-season sativa that produced great results when grown outdoors just inland from Monterey. The brothers grew in the mountains, where their crop was protected from the wind but still received the tremendous amount of light needed to develop big buds. When mature, their plants were very tall, between 6-12 feet, with long, thin buds that developed wispy red pistils. The aroma of the dried buds and smoke was complex and sweet, and the high it produced was very intense and cerebral with a psychedelic edge. Known as the Haze, this variety became popular in the Bay Area of California during the next decade.

The Haze Brothers eventually retired, but first they made a visit to the Netherlands, where they met with Nevil, a breeder whose name has often been associated with the Haze and its hybrids. Nevil acquired Haze seeds from them, preserving the strain and using it for many crosses. He found that pure Haze was a difficult variety to grow, requiring professional care and a lot of patience because of its long season, but it was very good for hybridization. Today, the Haze variety appears in many crosses that are available, and remains a favorite of many sativa connoisseurs.

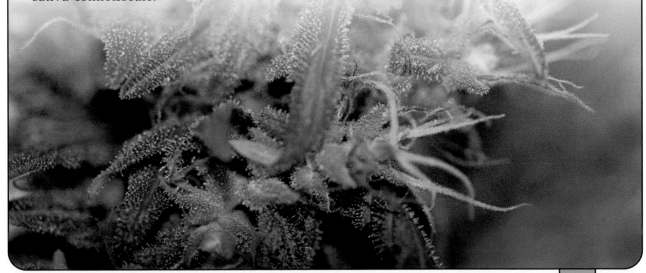

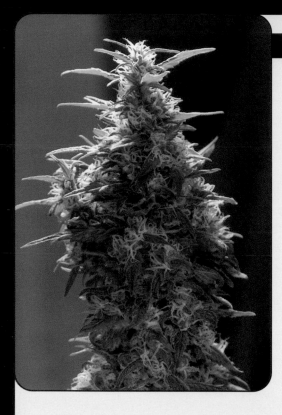

Haze 19 x Skunk #1

 IS 60/40

 63-70 days

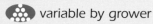

variable by grower

Haze 19 x Skunk #1

cerebral

fruity/citrus

This cross combines the famed Haze with Skunk #1 for a plant with a better yield and shorter finishing time than the full-blooded Haze, while still giving a soft fruity taste and sativa feeling.

A 60/40 indica sativa hybrid, this variety does well using any of the common indoor growing methods, including hydroponics and soil. Perfect for the impatient sativa lover, Haze 19 x Skunk #1 finishes in just 9-10 weeks with a satisfying yield and a mind expanding high. A great summertime weed, it is alert, sometimes even a little speedy.

The taste of this variety has been softened from the trademark haze and skunk flavors to a subtle but predominantly floral scent with just a whiff of the skunk. The moderate to high yield produces chunky nugs at multiple nodes. As with most Haze hybrids, this plant will get tall. Height consideration may encourage a shorter vegetative phase. Cultivating Haze 19 x Skunk #1 requires some plant intuition in determining vegetative and flowering times, making this a better variety for the green thumb or experienced grower.

Winner, *High Times* Cannabis Cup, 1992 for the Homegrown Fantasy coffeeshop

Huron

 75/25

 mid to late Sep

 Niagara x White Widow

 body relaxation

earthy/sweet

150-200 g per plant

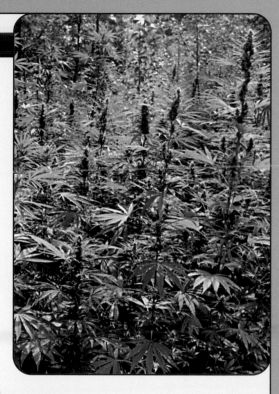

This cross of Dr. Greenthumb's flagship breed, Niagara, and the famed White Widow was developed with the outdoor grower in mind. Called Huron to honor its Canadian home, this strain was selected based on potency and an early finishing time.

Huron is a great outdoor plant for temperate latitudes, including most of Canada, Europe and the northern U.S. The best outdoor environment is in deep fertile soil, where it finishes by late September. Huron has survived the ultimate frost resistance test: unexpected snowfall, although handling frost is stronger in spring than autumn.

A good plant for the beginning grower, Huron can also be grown indoors when an outdoor garden is not possible. This plant will adapt well to most indoor methods and finish between 18-24 inches (45-60 cm). Dr. Greenthumb recommends pruning radially, then grouping out four branches for a multi-staked plant.

A three-quarter indica, this plant has a short stature and fat dense colas. The resin production makes some nice sticky buds, but the flower structure has an overall sativa feel to it. Huron has an earthy smell while growing as well as when dried, and the taste is still earthy but has some sweet tones also.

Huron fans swear by its medical usefulness, claiming it is great for pain relief, and offers a consistent, relaxing high that has a long duration.

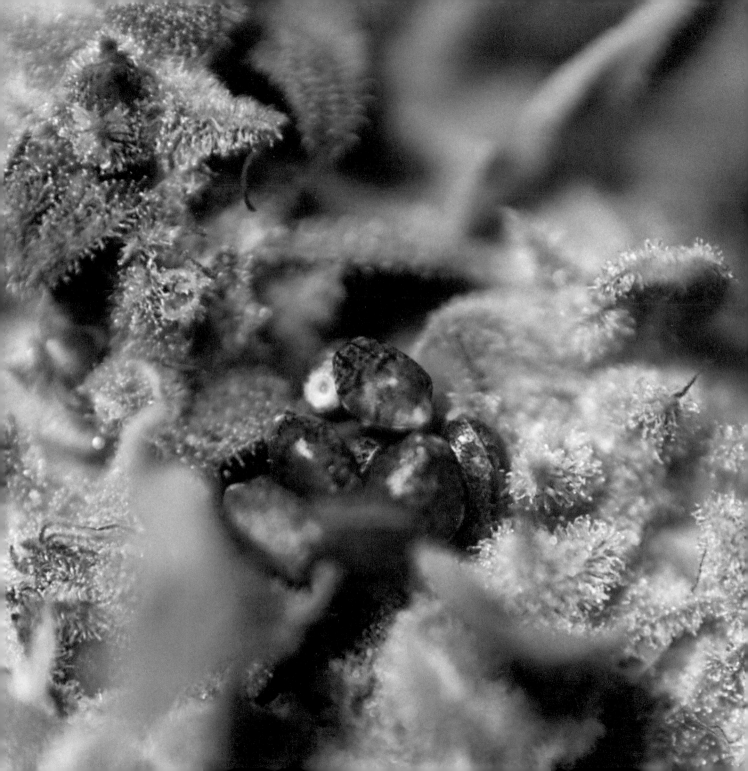

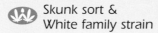

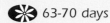 63-70 days

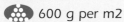

 600 g per m2

SOG

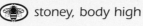 Skunk sort & White family strain

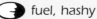 stoney, body high

fuel, hashy

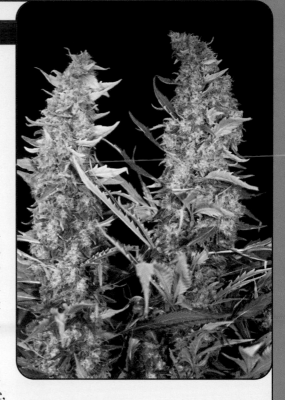

Two types of grass gained popularity among Dutch growers in the mid-1990s. The red skunk strains gave high yields of middling quality weed, while the resinous white strains satisfied any ganja gourmet with flavor and quality of buzz, but gave only modest yields. After an intense selection process, Nirvana hybridized for the best qualities of these two established strains with Ice.

A new generation power plant, Ice weds kind bud with kind yields. Ice has few branches, minimal foliage, and many floral clusters: a plus when manicuring. Virtually all of the branches Ice extends will be heavily budded. A rapid grower, this plant can be put directly into flower after roots are established. She will double in height and start forming flowers in the first 2 weeks of the 12 hour light regimen. No ice maiden, this strain is happiest with lots of fresh, warm humid air circulating around her. Hydroponic methods will give the most effective results with the best resin production. A sea of green set-up is appropriate.

Ice practically fumes with the nearly fuel-like scent of raw THC. Flavored like Nepali black hash, toking Ice is likely to induce coughing. Plan on putting your brain on ice because this variety's heavy stone may leave you in a lazy daze for hours.

Winner, *High Times* Cannabis Cup 1998

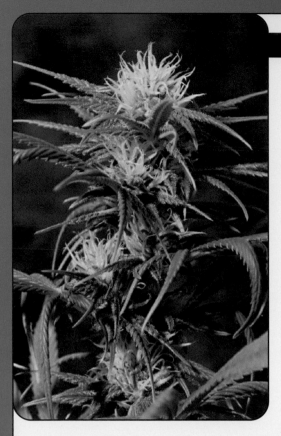

Island Sweet Skunk

 50-55 days

 2 oz. per plant in 1lb. per plant out

 Skunk #1

 mellow, cerebral

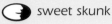 sweet skunk

SOG

I sland Sweet Skunk came to Federation by way of expat Vietnam veterans who settled on Vancouver Island in western Canada. The parent is a 1970s California Skunk #1 strain which was referred to as "Sweet Skunk." Stabilized outdoors, Island Sweet Skunk remains Federation's most prolific variety with outdoor yields averaging a pound per plant.

Island Sweet Skunk takes 8 weeks to finish in its Canadian home, but this variety can be ready to harvest after 7 weeks when grown at a higher altitude. The fluffy buds allow for good air flow, which reduces the chance of mold. Rain is easily dispersed and a little breeze leaves the colas dry and healthy. As it matures, these buds become covered with elongated orange-yellow hairs.

A real jumper in growth, Island Sweet Skunk will double in size when put into flowering indoors. A pole-straight growth pattern and minimal lateral branching make it possible to place plants close together in a sea of green set-up. The large main colas at the end of each plant give a great yield, even in small spaces, but should be staked. After vegetating for 2 months outdoors, this plant has reached heights of 12 feet, with a 3 pound yield that practically broke the branches off.

The Mission of Federation Seed Company

The Federation Seed Company took its name from a Gene Roddenberry–inspired universal view of a future with no war, hunger or poverty. We believe this future can be achieved, and have dedicated our life's endeavors to realizing this dream and turning it into reality. From space, the Earth is a teeny, tiny little blue pearl of life in a vast inkiness of cold, sterile blackness so immense it's hard to wrap your mind around it. Each and every one of us need to be responsible custodians of this Spaceship Earth for it holds the future of our species as a jumping-off point to the stars and beyond.

Federation Seed Company would like to see pot taken to outer space. We need to consider cannabis as a viable resource that we can and should take with us. Cannabis has so many applications, from lubricant to food to building materials, that make it an ideal plant of the new frontier.

Seeding the galaxy one planet at a time, the Federation Seed Company has one prime directive here on Earth—legalize cannabis around the globe. Federation's body of work can be found in the genetics we have bred and maintained over the years, and we sincerely hope they have contributed to a better m-class planet. All our eggs are in one basket and the future is depending on us to do the right thing. Live Long and Prosper,

Professor Ziggy

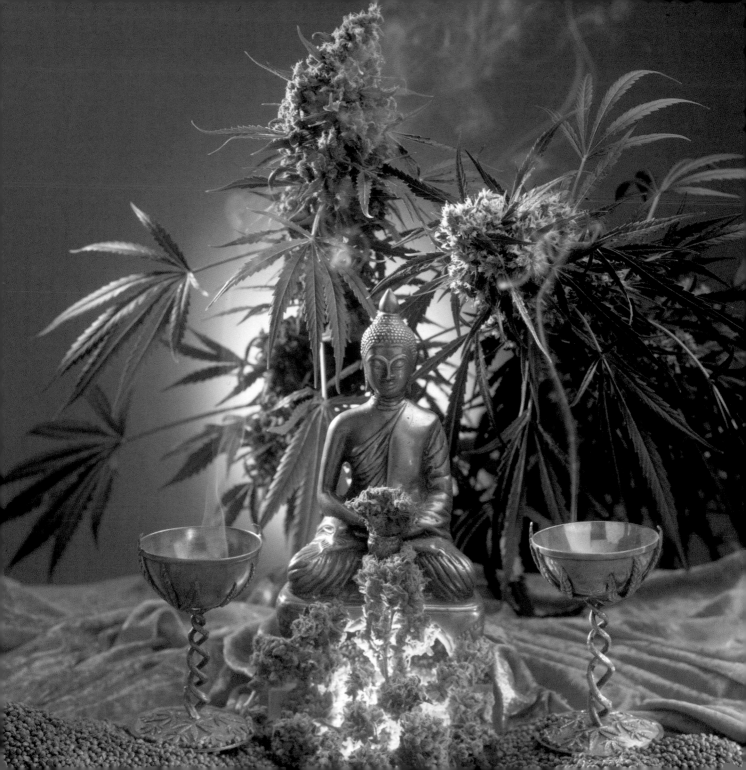

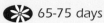

Jack Herer

 65-75 days

 450 g per m2

 Secret multiple hybrid Haze x Red Skunk strain

 cerebral, up

fresh, peppery

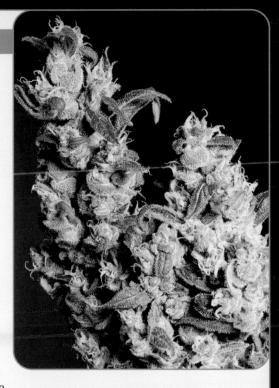

Named for beloved pot author and activist (see next page), Sensi's Jack Herer is truly one of the top hybrids ever created at the Cannabis Castle. The goal was to make a 50 percent Haze cross that kept the properties of this top-rated sativa, while shortening the painful 6 month flowering time that a full-blooded Haze demands.

This variety's long-fingered leaves and dense, grape-cluster bud formations appear light green due to the frosty resin coating. The few hairs on the buds turn brick red as the plant matures. The smell is fresh with a signature Haze accent and a pleasing hint of skunkiness. Since the rooted clones can go directly into flowering, the total number of light hours in the life cycle is almost exactly the same as a conventional indica-heavy cross, even though the flowering cycle is longer.

If growing in soil, full ground is recommended over pots, which are usually too small. Dry climates, like Spain and California are Jack Herer's only reasonable candidates for an outdoor home. Growing Jack indoors is necessary in most parts of the world. Hydroponics will give quick satisfying results, but Jack Herer is best grown as bigger plants.

A longer-flowering cross can be unnerving to grow, but bravery and patience will be rewarded with fresh peppery buds that produce an immediate cerebral, up high. Don't cave to the temptation and harvest too early. When allowed its full time to ripen, Jack Herer is a tasty smoke with mild lung expansion and possibly visually enhancing or silly effects.

Winner, *High Times* Cannabis Cup 1995

Jack Herer: Father of the New Hemp Industry

In 1973, some college students told Jack that marijuana was used in the old days as paper, fiber and canvas. Intrigued, Jack and his friend, Captain Ed, began researching hemp. Then in 1975, while tripping on acid, "All the millions of hemp facts came together in one huge realization: HEMP CAN SAVE THE WORLD!"

Jack says he and Captain Ed made a pledge "to work every day for the rest of our lives, or until we turned 84, to get pot legalized and free pot prisoners." That was 50 years away. Captain Ed died in 1991.

In 1981, Jack started handing out a 4-page essay on hemp that grew to 6 pages in 1983, and continued to expand when in 1986, Jack printed and handed out 50,000 copies as a tabloid newspaper. This 1986 copy contained the essay which was titled for the first time "The Emperor Wears No Clothes."

On the campaign trail ever since, Jack's "Emperor" is now in its 11th edition and is available worldwide in several languages. In 1989, after finding that the Smithsonian Museum in Washington D.C. had obliterated hemp from history, Jack obtained a permit and set up an alternative museum that was open 24 hours a day, 60 yards from the museum's entrance. It contained hemp objects including Bibles, canvas and a continuous loop of the movie, *Hemp for Victory,* that he had rescued from planned obscurity. This protest led to national publicity for the book, and for hemp and its main apostle.

Jack Herer is proof that a single person with a good idea can make a difference. After a century and a half of decline, the hemp industry has been reborn. He has ensured that 300 million people know about hemp's future.

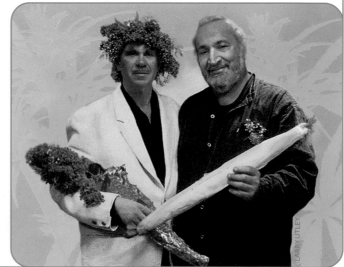

Jack Herer (right) and Ed Rosenthal (left) at Ed's Roast 'N Ball, hosted by Cannabis Action Network in 1999.

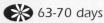

Kahuna

 63-70 days

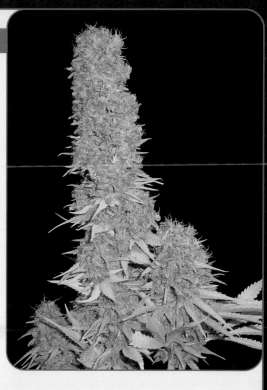

Super Skunk x
Big Skunk Korean x
Jack Herer x
Afghani Hawaiian

 alert, cerebral

25-30 g per plant in
1 gal. pot

 sweet/peppery

SOG

One of Soma's favorite strains, Kahuna is a 4-way cross that brings together a wide set of influences for a complex high. Soma recently renamed his Soma #9 strain Kahuna, which is a Hawaiian title for a religious or spiritual leader that literally means "Keeper of the Secret." The Kahuna variety has both tropical influences in its parentage, and spiritually attuning effects when used.

A medium-sized plant, Kahuna produces few side branches and a top bud that will impress you with its length and density. Due to the big, tight buds, conditions must be tended carefully for this variety. For indoor gardens, attention to humidity levels is key for mature buds that are mold-free. While recommended for indoors where variables can be controlled, outdoor growing is possible in reliably dry climates. An unseasonably rainy season could ruin the promising look of these thick buds with insidious mold.

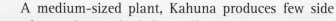

When Kahuna's proper conditions are met, the yield potential is fantastic, offering a harvest of up to 500 grams per square meter in a standard sea of green. This variety has shaken a little pepper into an otherwise sweet-tasting puff. A very sweet smelling variety with a powerful cerebral high that invites creativity, this is great daytime pot, complementary to most introspective activities, and comfortable for socializing with colleagues and friends. Kahuna offers medicinally valuable properties for many conditions without interfering with quality and clarity of one's thought.

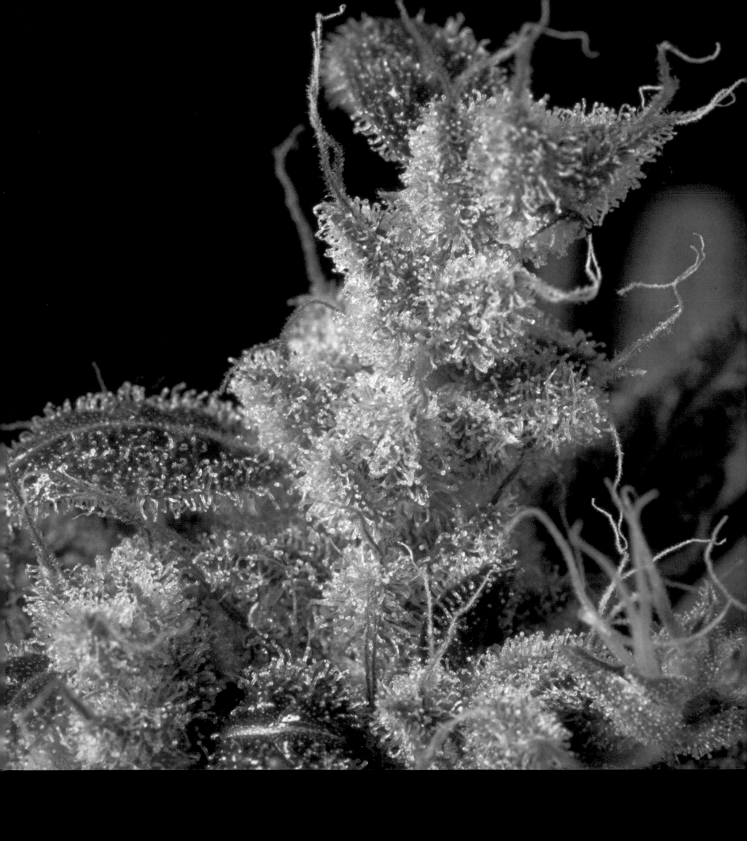

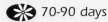
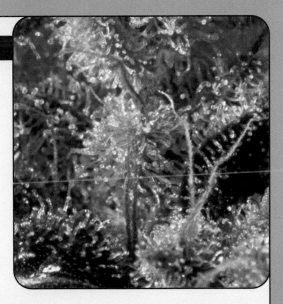

 S 80/90

❋ 70-90 days

SOG: 15-35 g per plant in; 300-500 g per plant out

 2 sativa dominant hybrids

 cerebral, energetic

sweet/spicy

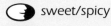 SOG

Kali Mist was developed in the early 1990s, when many primo sativas from mysterious origins were gathered and selectively bred. Kali has had a series of fathers, creating slight differences based on time period. Seeds first sold under this name strongly resembled the typical Southeast Asian sativa, but an interim father in the 1990s gave the offspring a more Afghani look. With the new millennium, Kali's third father has returned it to a strongly sativa appearance.

Kali plants grow to a medium height with long internodes and medium-long fan leaves. The plant's structure is "open," meaning it's possible to see all the way through the space between the plants. This structure promotes good quality buds along the entire length of the stem because light can penetrate through the entire plant. Big individual flowers cluster closely together to form buds that are mostly leafless in 75 percent of the plants. The other quarter form a more traditional bud with many leaflets. On both types, glandular trichomes abound.

Seedlings are ready to flower after 30-40 days of vegetative growth, when they should be clipped to avoid ungainly heights. Clones are ready for flowering as soon as they are rooted, about 3-4 days. Indoor growing is recommended, by any method, including sea of green. Kali can be attempted outside where long growing seasons prevail.

With a sweet scent and flavor that spans both the sweet and spicy, this variety offers a cerebral high that leaves the mind clear and focused. Kali Mist's effects have proven beneficial for medical users with multiple sclerosis, fatigue and chronic pain. A popular choice among women, Kali Mist is a great all-day pot that can enhance energetic outdoor activities or more meditative, thoughtful pastimes.

1st place, *High Times* Cannabis Cup hydro division 1995

1st place, *High Times* Cannabis Cup sativa category 2000

In 1994, Les and Cheryl Mooring were busted for growing 257 marijuana plants behind their barn in Clinton, Arkansas. Two registered and legally, owned pistols on top of their refrigerator increased the mandatory minimum sentences they faced to 25 and 15 years, respectively, in addition to the seizure of their property. In 1995, the Moorings fled prosecution, settling into a small town in the Netherlands where they started their lives over in exile, but not for long.

In an attempt to negotiate their case, the Moorings remained in contact with their probation officer. These calls lead to their location being identified and a request for their extradition to the U.S. They were picked up by Dutch authorities in November 1996.

Extradition requires the condition of "double criminality" to be met. This means that the offense must be punishable by imprisonment of at least one year under the laws of both states involved. Despite the commonly held belief that marijuana is legal in the Netherlands, possession of marijuana remains a punishable offense in the Dutch criminal code. In practice, marijuana is tolerated in the Netherlands—this "crime" would have resulted in plant confiscation, a fine, and possibly a period of community service. Regardless of this fact, the letter of the law allowed for extradition.

Many Americans and Dutch recognized the absurdity of the case, and organized in Holland to protest. Known as the Green Prisoners Release Organization, these activists began meeting at a canal house in Amsterdam that was managed by Henk Poncin. While the Moorings were returned to the United States in January 1997, the actions of this group helped bring attention to their case. On return, Cheryl Mooring, who had never smoked marijuana, was released with probation for failure to report a felony. Les Mooring was sentenced to serve 10 years.

After the Mooring case, the Green Prisoners group redirected their energy to the creation of a cannabis information center. Members from the Green Prisoners invested money and work into their vision, renovating the 17th century monument house that had become their headquarters thanks to Henk Poncin. The renovation, including a live cannabis garden built for educational purposes, was completed and Cannabis College opened its doors in 1998. It immediately met with an unexpected obstacle—the city of Amsterdam would not issue a permit allowing Cannabis College to sell any products. With all the funds for the project invested in the renovation, the founders had to rethink their approach or face the loss of all the hard work put into its formation.

In order to keep Cannabis College operational, they approached a well-known and reputable breeder, Eddy, of Flying Dutchmen. Eddy became involved in Cannabis College as a way of giving back to the plant he had been working with and earning a living from for 30 years. With his assistance, the College was able to open and maintain operations as a free public information center dedicated to cannabis.

The primary goal of Cannabis College is educational. Information is available on the many uses of this plant, including historical and medicinal as well as recreational uses of cannabis, and the almost limitless uses for hemp. Along with the exhibits, about 10 enthusiastic volunteers, who comprise the staff at Cannabis College, are happy to offer information and advice, direct visitors to resources, and lead tours of the garden. Visitors include tourists, locals, politicians, police and parents alike.

The world is engaged in a discussion about the fate of marijuana, and the founders and volunteers at Cannabis College are passionate about providing accurate and objective information for use in this dialog. Ultimately, Cannabis College hopes to branch out to other locations in Europe and North America, making accurate information on this plant as widespread as possible. The College is free and open to the public, so be sure to include a stop at this unique institution when in Amsterdam. If you can't make it in person, pay a virtual visit on the Web at www.cannabiscollege.com.

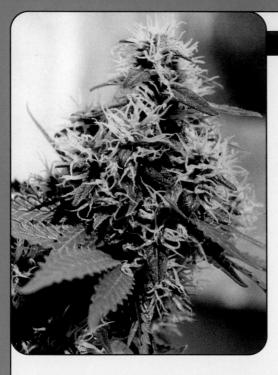

KC 33

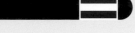

 60/40

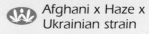 Afghani x Haze x Ukrainian strain

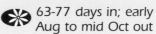 63-77 days in; early Aug to mid Oct out

 cerebral

 out preferred

lemon citrus

 up to 900 g per plant

A Dutch breed with Afghani and Eastern European progenitors, KC 33 got her name by way of the breeder's age in 1993 when she was developed. KC received the parent Afghani strain from a friend who had adapted the strain over 29 years of growing in the Netherlands. This was crossed with a Haze and another early flowering plant from the Ukraine. The result is a plant that can finish in Holland as early as August and as late as October outdoors, depending on the time it is planted.

KC 33 was developed with the outdoor grower in mind, but can be grown indoors as a large plant with a yield of up to 600 g using 600 wpm. A sea of green method is discouraged. Outdoors, she loves moisture and will thrive even in cool, wet weather. The Haze and Ukrainian parents are known to reach gigantic heights. Inheriting this height, KC 33 can be planted later in the season than is customary to steer clear of her leggy qualities while still bringing in a generous yield before the first frost. Alternately, outdoor growers can use a covering system to reduce light hours and finish plants when most gardens are just entering flowering phase. The stretchy height has also been put to use by trellising this variety and growing horizontally.

KC 33 has enormous leaves and enormous sweet, sticky, light green buds with a distinctive lemon taste that is fresh on the palate. Smoking KC 33 results in a light unencumbered buzz that settles into the head instead of the body.

La Niña

  75/25  Haze x White Widow

 56-70 days in Sep out creeper

spicy fruit

450-550 g per m2

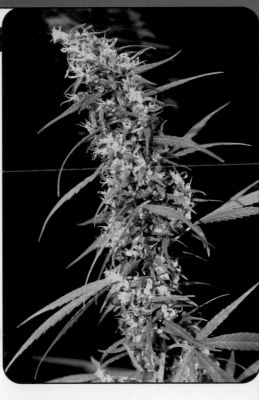

After years of being held in reserve for family members, La Niña became available to the general public in 1998.

Strongly related to El Niño, La Niña manifests characteristics that are predictable, contrary to her name's implication.

A three-quarter sativa, La Niña is a good selection for the Haze lover, but not as good for a beginner's garden. Indoor growing requires meticulous trimming and an early force into flower to control the Haze-influenced size. This plant can touch the sky if not kept trimmed. While requiring a decent outdoor growing season, a finishing time of 8-10 weeks is getting off pretty easy for a Haze fan. The finish will be on the earlier side if you reside in an equatorial region.

La Niña's buds are large and airy like the Haze, and produce thick crystals which tend to have a shorter neck and bigger head than most glands. As it finishes, La Niña barely looks like a pot plant, more resembling a Spanish broom plant because the flowers are so long and airy. The exotic Haze flavor consisting of mild sweet fruity tones was a point of selection in this hybrid, and remains intact through the cross.

With La Niña around, life will never be tame again. The high is so clear, you might feel seduced into thinking that you're sober . . . until you try to do things, and feel the electricity of the buzz in your actions.

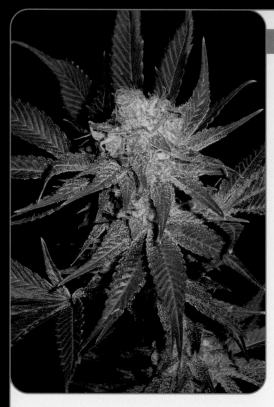

Lavender

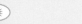

 56-63 days

 Super Skunk x
Big Skunk Korean x
Afghani Hawaiian

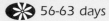

12-15 g per plant in
1 gal. pot

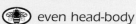 even head-body

spicy

Lavender brings together a world of weed. Strains with histories that traverse Afghanistan, Hawaii, Korea, the U.S., and Europe are all melded together in this 3-way cross. An exotic looking strain, Lavender develops the darkest purple coloration you can imagine. The color is intense, with the leaves turning nearly to black at the ends, they are so deeply saturated with color. The extra dense buds give off a sensually spicy smell akin to Afghani hash.

The high calyx-to-leaf ratio and the legginess of this plant make for simplified manicuring. While not as tall as the Haze strains, Lavender can shoot to tall heights when allowed an extended vegetation period before being placed into the flowering phase. If grown in a sea of green, Soma recommends shortening the veg cycle in order to control the height. This strain will also do well as a multi-branched plant. Outdoors, this variety can thrive in most temperate zones, although arid climates known for their rich agricultural promise are of course optimal.

Lavender has a flavor that is similar to Afghani hash, producing a captivating high that circulates through every chakra. A terrific evening or rainy day smoke, Lavender will leave you feeling relaxed and mellow, possibly to the point of sleep.

How Soma Started Out:

"In 1971, I was living in Vermont, and I used to roll seeded weed all the time, and at that time, seeds were just something I didn't want to smoke. I was always taking a record album and sorting the seeds out of the bud. I lived on the second floor, and all winter I was throwing the seeds out the window. In the springtime, when I went outside, I noticed that alongside the house there were all these little baby cannabis plants sprouting from the seeds I'd been throwing out there. I didn't even start growing on purpose, but when I saw these live plants growing from the seeds, I just had this instant urge to transplant them into nicer pots and take them to a nicer spot. And that's how I started growing cannabis, kind of by pure accident.

Well, the seeds I was trying to grow were a sativa strain from Colombia—like a pure sativa strain. And here I was growing in the cold climate of Vermont, outdoors, and this strain could never finish before it froze. I didn't know any better at the time. I'd just started, but that was my first insight into breeding. I could see this breed wasn't suitable for the area where I was growing it. I started thinking about selection: basically how could I come up with a strain that would be suitable for the area where I lived. Some friends of mine had been in Afghanistan, which is also a cold climate, and they brought some seeds back. I got a hold of some of those seeds and started growing pure Afghani, which did do well outdoors in Vermont and could finish soon enough. I started experimenting, crossing that strain with other ones, and then it just kept expanding. Now I work with 51 different mother plants. I have about 75 different kinds of seeds. I basically have every type of genetic represented, from Southeast Asian to pure Afghanis, in those 51 mothers."

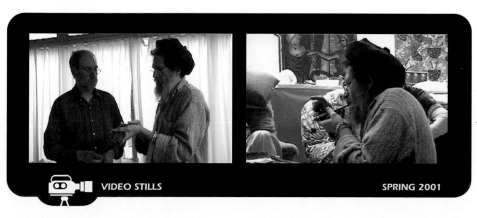

Hanging out with Soma at his pad in Amsterdam

VIDEO STILLS   SPRING 2001

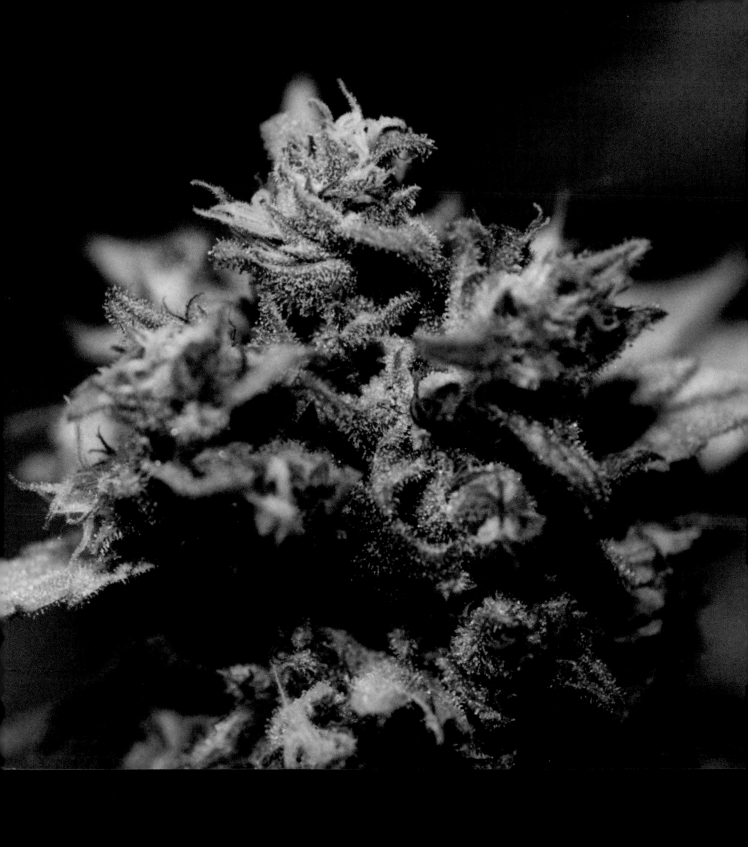

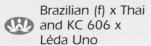

Léda Uno

SI 60/40

49-63 days in 77 days or mid-Sep out

out preferred

20-100 g per plant in; 2-3 kilos per plant out

Brazilian (f) x Thai and KC 606 x Léda Uno

body stone, giggly

lemon citrus

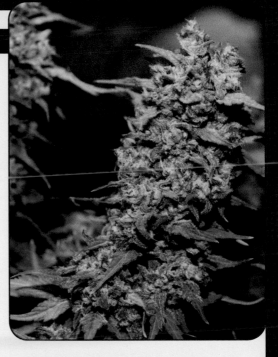

Léda Uno acquired her mysterious Brazilian name directly from a South American woman named Léda who risked bringing male pollen from a Brazilian plant to KC in Holland. The pollen was dusted on a hybrid of Brazilian/Thai female crossed with KC 606.

Specially designed by KC Brains for outdoor gardening, Léda Uno should not be shied away from by indoor gardeners who prefer larger plants. Indoors or out, this lady likes arid weather and can stand very dry periods without difficulties. Moist weather may introduce problems, so consider the humidity levels and rain in the growing season of your region before committing to an outdoor grow with this variety. When grown in amenable European climates, a 3 month cycle from start to finish will produce a plant that is upwards of 12 feet (4.5 meters) tall, making this plant obvious to passersby if size is not controlled. However, a plant grown to this proportion can yield up to 2-3 kilos. Inside yields can vary between 20-100 g per plant under 400-600 watts of light, depending on the grower's method, ability and harvesting time.

A 60 percent sativa, Léda Uno is tall and sleek, with finger-like leaves and a sweet lemon aroma. The buds are fat indica-type colas. The taste is like a lemon drop, without the tangier tones that lemon sometimes evokes. While still growing, these plants exude a fresh aroma and appear sugar-coated with glands. The champagne of ganjas, Léda Uno can be bubbly and psychedelic, a sociable intelligent buzz. In greater amounts, however, she may leave you locked on the couch with your tongue tied and eyelids at half-mast.

2nd place, *High Life* Cannabis Cup 1998

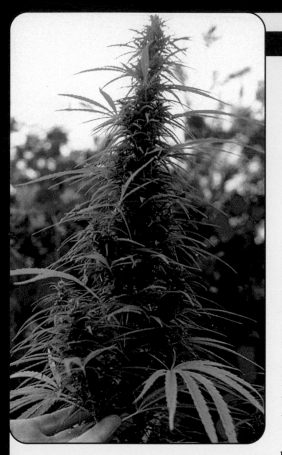

Malawi Gold

 S

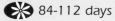 84-112 days

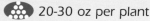 20-30 oz per plant

 Sativa from the Salima region, Malawi

 psychoactive with clarity

 sweet, floral, pineapple

Malawi Gold is the quintessential sativa, with large slim fan leaves that often become very dark in color. These plants like to grow tall, and branch heavily, and may develop reddish-purple coloration as they mature. The structure is pyramidal, much like a Christmas tree. Malawi Gold likes to grow large with multiple branches, all of which will yield some lovely buds.

As an equatorial sativa, the maturation time is considerable, but the resulting buds are sticky, with visible resin glands. Outdoors, buds can grow up to 2 feet long. The smell is pleasantly sweet and refreshing, while the smoke is slightly bitter with pineapple and almond aftertastes. The buzz has an enjoyably alert mental clarity, but is very psychoactive and the high is long lasting.

Malawi Gold is well known as some of the best and finest sativa from Africa. In Malawi, the buds are cured after being tightly bound in banana leaf to give a compact, potent gold-colored product. This variety is grown outdoors in several regions of Malawi, where it can range in size from 6-12 feet depending on the conditions and growing time. Malawi Gold likes warm climates with daytime temperatures over 80 degrees F and 5 months minimum frost free periods. Germination is improved by matching this plant's native conditions.

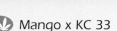

 I

 42-63 days in
63-77 days out

 out preferred

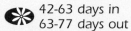 4-5 kilos per plant

 Mango x KC 33

 body stone

 mango, sweet

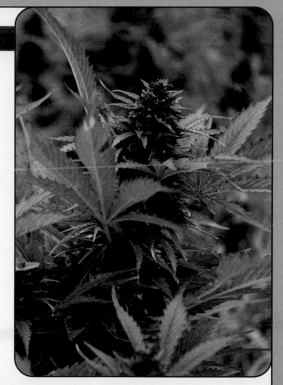

Mango's parentage is part KC 33 and part Mango from a hippie fellow who grew it for 30 years, then let KC use it as a cross in 1991. This variety is a 100 percent indica strain that grows large and produces prodigiously.

Don't let Mango's slow start fool you—this variety will eventually rival the impressive size of many KC varieties, which are especially intended for outdoor grows. If you want Mango to stay at an average size in an outdoor garden, allow only 3 weeks of vegetative time and transplant outdoors as late as July in Northern latitudes. Mango can also be grown in an indoor garden, but needs a lot of space. If you want some monster indoor plants, allow seedlings or clones to vegetate for 3-4½ weeks before changing to a 12/12 light regimen. Mango gardeners must rule with an iron fist if they want to manage the size of this plant, and it is important to start the discipline early. Accomplish this by starting the flowering phase about 1½ – 2 weeks after the seedling has sprouted and proven vigorous. Once established, Mango plants will grow so fast, you can practically watch them change height before your eyes.

Mango buds are massive and weighty, growing to lengths of 18 inches and the circumference of a woman's calf. Luckily the branches give sturdy support. As it matures, this plant's foliage can turn a very red to reddish purple color. The smell and taste are decidedly sweet mango and the stone is an even, mellow body sensation.

Pot in Canada: The Early Days
■ Dana Larsen

Cannabis has been grown on Canadian soil since 1609, when Louis Hebert, a successful Parisian apothecary and friend of explorer Samuel de Champlain, harvested his first crop of cannabis and other plants in Nova France (now Nova Scotia). Skilled in the use of plant medicines, it is certain that Hebert was well aware of the medicinal properties of his cannabis buds.

Cannabis remained a staple crop in Canada until the early 1920s, when anti-pot sentiment began spreading across North America. In Canada, the flames of prohibition were fanned by Emily Murphy. Renowned as a champion for women's rights, Murphy was also a harsh racist who wrote under the pen name of "Janey Canuck."

Her most famous book, *The Black Candle*, was a very biased and sensationalized diatribe against cannabis and opium that was serialized in *Maclean*'s magazine. In one chapter, a Los Angeles County Chief of Police is quoted as saying that:

"Persons using this narcotic smoke the dry leaves of the plant, which has the effect of driving them completely insane. The addict loses all sense of moral responsibility. Addicts to this drug, while under its influence are immune to pain, and could be severely injured without having any realization of their condition. While in this condition they become raving maniacs and are liable to kill or indulge in any form of violence to other persons, using the most savage methods of cruelty without, as said before, any sense of moral responsibility."

Throughout much of the book, Ms. Murphy uses race to inflame, claiming that "Chinese peddlers" and "Negroes coming into Canada" were engaged in a menacing plan to rule the world by getting the white race hooked on

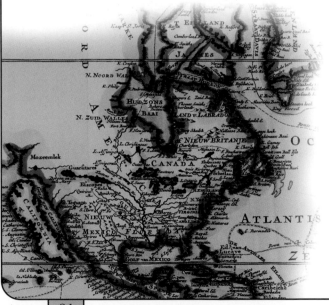

"dope," which they knew better than to use themselves.

When *The Black Candle* was released in 1922, its sole purpose was to arouse public opinion and pressure the government into creating stricter drug laws. The Royal Canadian Mounted Police used this book to increase its power along with making cannabis illegal under the name "marijuana" in the Opium and Narcotic Drug Act of 1923.

In 1954 possession for the purpose of trafficking was created as a new offense in Canada, with a sentence of seven years. The sentence for this crime was immediately doubled in the following year, raising the maximum penalty to fourteen years imprisonment.

The Single Convention on Narcotic Drugs took effect in 1961. While this Act eliminated whipping as a remnant of the anti-Chinese days, it also increased the minimum penalty for cultivation of marijuana or opium poppies to seven years, and that for importation and exportation to fourteen years. Marijuana now carried the second heaviest minimum sentence in Canadian criminal law, surpassed only by sentencing for murder.

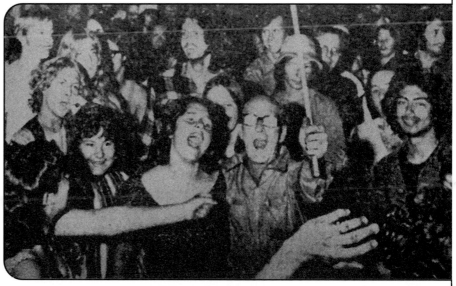

The crowd at Vancouver's Grasstown rally prior to police arrival.
courtesy "Cannabis Culture" magazine

Despite the draconian penalties, the 1960s saw marijuana use among Canadian youth become more widespread than ever before. The United States became embroiled in the Vietnam War, and many conscientious objectors avoided the draft by fleeing to Canada, where they grew pot to support themselves. Much of the famed BC Bud now exported to the U.S. comes from genetics first brought to Canada by these American draft-dodgers.

A crowd gathers for the Grasstown Smoke-In & Jamboree, 1971 courtesy "Cannabis Culture" magazine

By the late 1960s, the Canadian government seemed to be easing up on marijuana prohibition. Canada's Minister of Health and Welfare was quoted as saying that "both the Canadian and U.S. governments, by employing scare tactics, have been guilty of the indiscriminate overkill which has been effective only in reducing our own credibility."

The Le Dain Commission was appointed in Canada to undertake a complete and factual study of marijuana use and its effects. The results of the study were presented to the government in 1971, after four years and four million dollars' worth of research.

The Le Dain Commission recognized that the use of marijuana is not linked to violent crime in any way. It also concluded that prohibitionist laws have only served to create a subculture with little respect for the law and law enforcement, as well as diverting law enforcement capability, clogging the judicial system, and providing a base of funds for organized crime. The recommendations of the Le Dain Commission ranged from outright legalization to small fines for marijuana use.

After the commission's recommendations were announced, a "smoke-in" was held in Vancouver's Gastown. The event was called Grasstown, and attracted a few hundred activists, hippies and curious onlookers. Although this event began well, with songs being sung and a twenty-foot joint being passed around, the chief of police at this time felt the demonstration was a flagrant violation of law that could not be tolerated, and mounted policemen stormed the event, followed by the riot squad. Many of the event's participants suffered injuries, as did innocent bystanders and local shopkeepers who did not identify themselves quickly enough.

By the late 1970s there seemed to be consensus in parliament that marijuana needed to be legalized. Many politicians of the time, including Joe Clark, Pierre Trudeau, and Jean Chretien, publicly stated that they would enact some form of marijuana decriminalization as soon as possible. Unfortunately, the election of Ronald Reagan as President of the United States in 1980 ruined any chance of this happening.

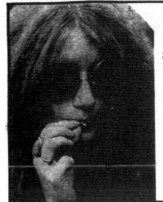

GRASSTOWN SMOKE-IN & STREET JAMBOREE

Smoking Marijuana is more fun than drinking beer but a friend of ours was captured and they gave him thirty years
Maybe we should raise our voices — ask somebody why but demonstrations are a drag — besides we're much too high.
And I'm sure it wouldn't interest anybody. . . . outside of a small circle of friends.
— Phil Ochs.

SATURDAY NIGHT 8:30 pm Maple Tree Square (WATER & CARRALL)

courtesy "Cannabis Culture" magazine

With Nancy Reagan at the helm, the U.S. War on Drugs began in earnest once again, and Canada dutifully went along with their Southern Neighbors.

Dana Larsen has served as editor of *Cannabis Culture* magazine since its inception in 1994. He has written hundreds of articles and essays on cannabis and drug policy, history and related issues. Dana is also a founding member of the BC and Canadian Marijuana Parties, and is the author of the *Pot Puzzle Fun Book*. *Cannabis Culture* can be accessed online at www.cannabisculture.com

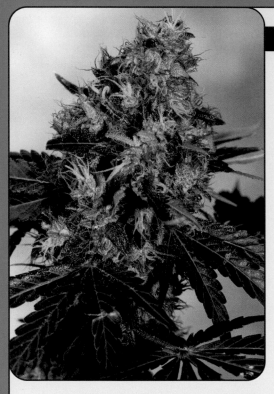

Mangolian Indica

 I

 55-60 days

 300-325 g per m2

 Afghani skunk x
Afghani x
Northern Lights

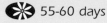 sleepy, physical

fresh woodsy scent/
mango citrus taste

Mangolia is not an exotic locale, but rather a made-up word to describe the citrus-mango flavor of this indica bud. Mangolian Indica's parents are from several genetic pools with origins in Afghanistan, making this a well-adapted plant for outdoor growing in temperate zones. It has been grown outdoors with good results in Holland.

Mangolian Indica stays fairly short, averaging 3 feet (1 meter) in height. The long slender foliage hints at some sativa in this hybrid, but the shrubby habit is all indica, and the heavy body stone leaves little doubt that this plant weighs in as a heavily indica cross. Flower tops have enough girth to yield over 300 grams per square meter, and are workable in most common indoor methods, including a sea of green, although the bushy nature requires some trim time to maximize light for the buds.

When growing, this strain smells very fresh and woodsy with a subtle skunk edge. The dried buds have a mango bouquet and a tasty citrus-mango flavor. The strong fruit taste will linger without turning to charcoal at the end of the joint. The Mangolian stone is long lasting and lethargic, with potential psychedelic dimensions—a perfect companion for a movie marathon or a lazy Sunday afternoon.

Master Kush

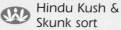

 63-70 days in end Oct out

 varies

SOG

Hindu Kush & Skunk sort

 body stone, visual

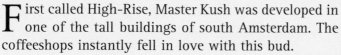 mildly earthy/citrus

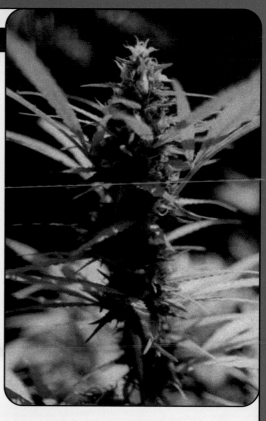

First called High-Rise, Master Kush was developed in one of the tall buildings of south Amsterdam. The coffeeshops instantly fell in love with this bud.

A vigorous plant, Master Kush thrives under most growing conditions, producing well in indoor and greenhouse set-ups. This variety grows into a medium-sized, compact, densely formed plant with sparse, spiky, forest green leaves. Master Kush's ball-shaped buds are light green with long hairs that range from white to orange in color. Buds are dense, thick, and heavy, which makes mold a risk in humid climates. Advantageously non-smelly while growing, the resulting bud has a hint of earthiness and sweet citrus but is virtually without taste.

Easy on lungs and palate, Master Kush is non-expansive and smooth to smoke, giving an all-over body buzz that is relaxing but awake. The high can also create optically pleasing effects, making it a good candidate for taking in a movie or museum visit.

Winner, *High Times* Cannabis Cup 1992
Winner, *High Times* Cannabis Cup 1993

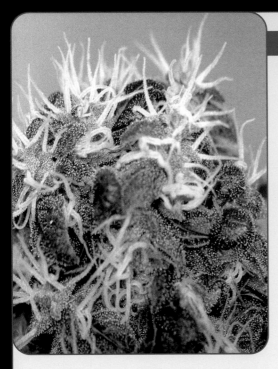

Matanuska Tundra

  Alaskan hybrid

 60-68 days in Oct out creepy, sleepy

 chocolate

In preferred

350-375 g per m2 in

Given to Sagarmatha from growers in the Matanuska Valley, this variety revives the majestic, legendary pot of the great Alaskan northland. This strain has also been known as Matanuska Thunderfuck, but Sagarmatha decided to use the more prudent "Tundra." As the Alaskan word for "grassland," Tundra makes this variety's name perfectly descriptive—it's grass from Alaska's grasslands!

Proven as a great stable breed for crossing, Matanuska Tundra has been widely used in Sagarmatha's hybrid programs. The flavor is chocolate, and the stone is a creeper, registering slowly and growing to a full, lethargic stone in the 5-10 minutes after a bong hit. Medical users have had good results alleviating pain with this variety.

An indica with enormous, palm-like leaves, Tundra stays short, but grows very thick with numerous side branches. Fat colas are coated with a frosty glacier of THC crystals. Sagarmatha recommends growing indoors. In an arid outdoor environment, this variety produces some chunky pot bushes that stay close to the ground and give good yields.

Gardeners should gauge Matanuska Tundra's ripeness by the lower portion of the buds because the tips of the top buds will keep growing when the rest of the bud is ripe. Waiting for the tips to finish can cause frustrating and unnecessary delays in harvesting. Sagarmatha breeders experimented with this phenomenon, waiting to harvest one plant until the tips finished.

After 115 days, they surrendered even though the top buds still had new, immature white hairs when they harvested. This plant must also be dried thoroughly because it may mold during the drying period if all of the moisture is not able to escape.

indica (m) x sativa (f)

 49 days in
mid-Sep out

 cerebral

 floral

500-550 g per m2
 with 600 wpm in
8-14 oz. per
unpruned plant out

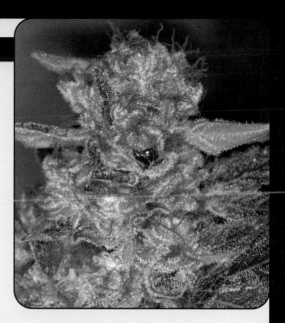

Max 49 was found in a tray of clones. When grown out, it showed more vigor and flowered earlier than its sisters. The buds were big tight fists running down the stem that were crammed with high potency glands.

Since discovered, Max 49 has been cloned extensively along North America's west coast. From it's characteristics, experts suggest that this plant was a cross of a male indica with a female sativa. Originally offered only as a clone for medical gardens, a female plant was masculinized over many years using a unique technique, then crossed back with itself to produce stable, all-female seeds.

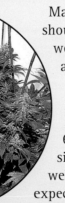

Max 49 is a short plant that branches extensively. In a sea of green, it should be pruned twice: once when entering flowering, and then again 2 weeks later. Using this method, Max 49 grows a single stem which acts as a platform for the strong, no-nonsense buds, that mature into a solid, $1\frac{1}{2}$-2 inch thick, foot-long column of densely packed flowers. At harvest, Max will reach a height of 30 inches (75 cm). When grown as larger plants indoors, Medifarm recommends trimming to one stem per 6-inch square. Outdoor plants grow about 3 feet (1 meter) with extensive branching, and need only moderately intense sunlight to mature well, although they will also thrive under bright sun. In warm climates, expect a smaller plant and an early finish.

Cured Max bud retains the floral sweet tones of the live plant, as does the taste. With cerebral, energetic and intense effects, Max 49 in moderation throughout the day produces an enjoyable yet focused high.

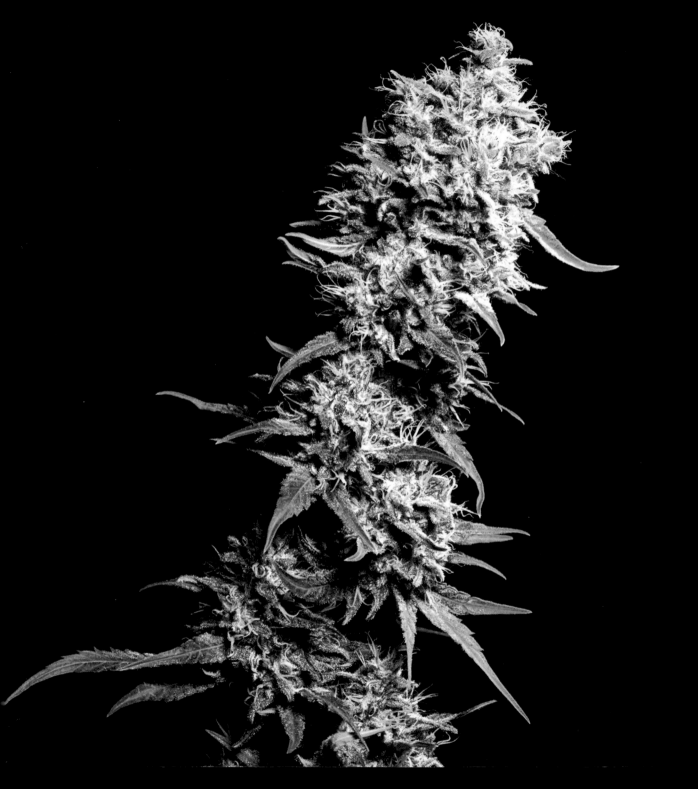

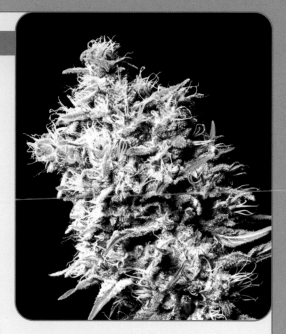

  S I

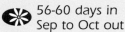 56-60 days in
Sep to Oct out

 Brazilian sativa x
South Indian x
Afghani

 up to 600 g per m2

 body stone

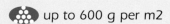 acrid, ripe fruit

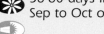 SOG

A proven medical marvel, Medicine Man is ideal for those in need of high THC levels. This variety has a strong heritage stemming from the Brazilian and South Indian genetics of White Widow crossed with a prodigious yielding Afghani. Sibling to the award-winning White Rhino, Medicine Man is indica in appearance, with a sturdy Christmas tree formation and immense crystal production.

Buds are dense and solid with yellow and red hairs. This variety changes color to silver as it finishes. Those who prefer to grow indoors can expect an incredibly resinous, compact plant. Outdoor gardeners will find that Medicine Man can get large outside and will get even stronger resin under natural sunlight. Medicine Man is not the easiest plant to get right but with love and attention, presents no real problems for the dedicated gardener. Mr. Nice Seed Bank recommends fertilizing conservatively for optimal results.

A proven champion for sick and terminally ill patients, the aptly named Medicine Man is serious stuff. Due to its heavy, sedating effect, you want to monitor your intake while toking, and especially when eating it in baked goods. This very strong, long-lasting buzz has proven effective for many conditions that benefit from cannabis, including anorexia, glaucoma, severe headaches, depression, AIDS and cancer/chemotherapy.

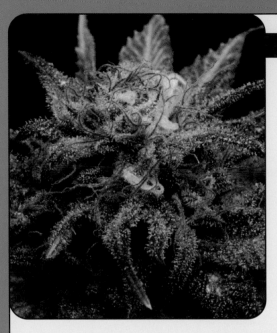

Mikado

 42-45 days in early Aug to mid-Sep out

 indica

 mellow body stone

 berry

1.5 oz per 2 gal. plant in; 1 lb per plant out

Mikado is a fast producing indica, finishing as early as August in temperate outdoor latitudes and as soon as 6 weeks indoors with desirable yields. A title for the emperor of Japan, the name Mikado is composed of the Japanese words "mi" (honorable) and "kodo" (gate of the imperial palace). Other interpretations give this term the meanings "God of the Sun" and "open August gate" in Japanese.

Federation developed this variety around 1993. Flavored like wild raspberries, this branchy variety develops purple leaves and calyxes during maturity. The buds are very fat and squat with distinctly pink hairs upon finish. Federation recommends growing Mikado indoors as a larger multi-branched plant, which suits the tendencies of this variety, leading to a better yield. Sea of green is less than optimal for this indica, since it likes to stay short and spread out. A terrific choice for outdoor growing, Mikado can yield a pound per plant and reduces work and worry with its early finish.

The Mikado high is a mellow body stone that is good for an evening smoke, especially when enjoying casual activities such as watching movies or chilling out with your friends.

Winner, Nimbin Cup 2000

IS 75/25

50 days

SOG: up to 400 g per m2 in; 300-400 g per plant out

SOG

Iranian Indica x (Niagara x Shiva)

strong body high, munchies

earthy, sweet, spicy

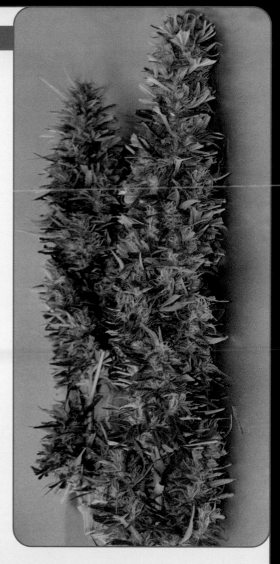

Dr. Greenthumb hand-selected the indica from the eastern mountains of Iran that dominates this hybrid. Millennium is balanced with a 25 percent cross of the sativa influenced Niagara/Shiva hybrid as second parent. An easy-to-grow variety indoors and out, Millennium was named with a hopeful look to its proliferation in the years to come.

This strain finishes in an average of 50 days with promising yield potential. The medium flower-to-leaf ratio makes this a manageable plant for a sea of green growing style, but it will also work as a staked multi-branch plant. When put into flowering at a foot tall, Millennium grows to a comfortable height of 24-30 inches (60-80 cm). Dr. Greenthumb recommends pinching off between the 4th and 5th node to save space and get 4 good, cola-producing branches. In the great outdoors, this plant reaches heights of 5-8 feet, and is a vibrant, vigorous grower in Canada and other temperate latitudes.

Millennium has a heavy hashy bouquet, but the flavor is earthy and sweet with sandalwood tones. This is not pot to smoke on your way into work, or when you are going to need to drive anywhere soon. Millennium offers a strongly physical, intense buzz for some couch potato time. Your refrigerator may also be subject to raiding when the munchies take hold.

Tony on Naming Sagarmatha:

"I had just come back from a trip through Nepal, and I was searching for a name for the company. There are different power points around the earth, and I think that Sagarmatha, which is the Nepalese name for Mt. Everest, is one of those sites. It's very inspiring. Sagarmatha translates to mean 'Sugar Mother.' The Everest glacier is the watershed for the valley, and so it's like a mother nurturing all the crops that are growing below. Well, I was thinking these nice sinsemilla colas—well, and the seeded ones too—they're all sugary coated, and they're all mamas, and they're giving you that good feeling. The name Sagarmatha, seemed like a really accurate choice, it tickled me for the layers of meaning. It's also a good, fun name because Sagarmatha is the highest place on earth. It's the tallest peak, and so we kind of joke around and think that some of our products are the highest you can get and still be on the ground."

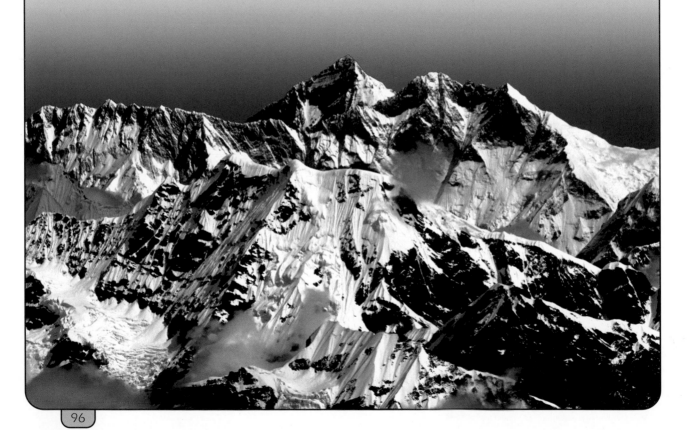

Nirvana

Nirvana means "a state of happiness." The history of Nirvana Seed Company goes back to the end of the 1980s, when the founder was working at Amsterdam's legendary "Positronics" growshop. The knowledge and inspiration he received there moved him to think about starting his own seed company. Years were spent traveling, seeking out and collecting seeds from the finest strains. More years went into experimentation, growing, cross breeding and developing the new strains from among which Nirvana selected the best to become their range of high quality hybrid seeds. After applying and expanding his experience in a number of Amsterdam's best known growshops, he opened Nirvana in 1995. An innovative business concept that developed into a full smart shop, Nirvana has a unique and original range of self-developed hemp products, that include hemp vinegar, hemp ice tea, and hemp liqueur as well as hemp wine and beer. Located in the heart of the picturesque Pijp, the Nirvana shop lives up to its name, adding color and serenity to the surrounding streets. Inside, among the holy images and products, the vibe is mellow and the staff is always happy to offer advice and suggestions, or just hang out.

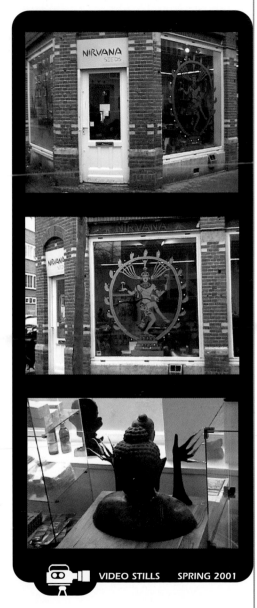

VIDEO STILLS   SPRING 2001

The Nirvana Shop (top and center)
Many religious sculptures grace the
shop's interior (bottom).

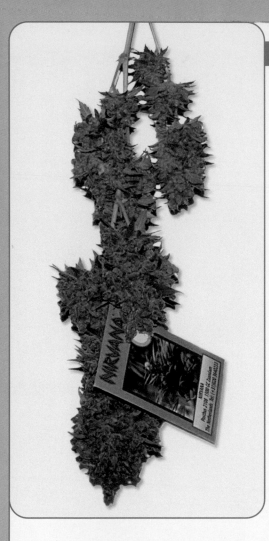

Misty

 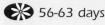

 56-63 days

 up to 500 g per m2

SOG

White Widow x
Northern Lights/
Shiva

 uplifting, social

 old sock

Misty is short and stocky, bringing out the indica side of the White family. The lime green, bubble-like leaves are thick and heavy like salad. Buds are dense and fat with THC glands extending to the shade leaves.

Highly recommended for a sea of green system, Nirvana suggests growing Misty plants close together in soil. Because they stay diminutive in size, you can pack a lot into a little space and finish with up to 500 grams per square meter. Misty is an indoor girl, and she likes her room kept cool and dry, preferably around 75 degrees F (24 degrees C) with 50 percent humidity.

This is musky pot, giving off a powerful smell that some say reeks of old sweat. Unlike its near offensive aroma, Misty smokes sweet and leaves a sugar after-taste in the mouth. Despite its rather indica appearance, the buzz retains a sativa influence, providing an uplifting and social experience. According to Amsterdam smokers, Misty joints seem to last longer than most, increasing their overall satisfaction ratings.

60-65 days

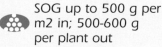
SOG up to 500 g per m2 in; 500-600 g per plant out

 White Widow & potent father

 cerebral, trippy

 fruity, sweet

 SOG

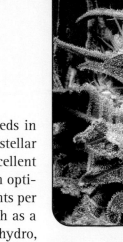

Nebula means starcloud. Bred by Paradise Seeds in 1996, this variety received the name for its stellar qualities. Nebula has an open structure that is excellent for indoor farming where the plants perform with optimal results in a sea of green set-up. Using 20 plants per square meter in this system, yields can be as high as a half-kilo. Not too finicky, Nebula will do well in hydro, coco or soil indoors. This variety has been successfully grown outdoors in Holland and would be an appropriate choice for outdoor gardens in temperate zones that offer a 9 week minimum flowering time before the first frost.

Nebula stretches slightly, but produces obesely fat buds when placed under lots of light. Like the name suggests, Nebula twinkles with the coating of THC glands, which are bound to take you into the realms of space—or possibly just make you spacy. The buzz is transcendental and cerebral, sometimes bordering on the psychedelic. Nebula may earn the nickname "honey pot" for it's sweet smell and distinctively honeyed fruit flavor. This variety is a fun tasty smoke, even for the veteran stoner.

4th place, *High Times* Cannabis Cup 1999
4th place, *High Times* Cannabis Cup 2000

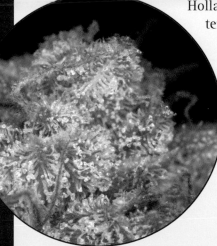

photo credit: Eric K and Paradise Seeds

Marijuana: World Traveler
▪ S. Newhart

Cannabis has long been a well-traveled plant. According to most accounts, the cannabis plant is originally from the foothills and mountain ranges that form the curving northern boundary of India from the Arabian Sea to the Bay of Bengal. This includes parts of India, Iran, the Hindu Kush region in Afghanistan and Pakistan, and the Himalayas in Nepal.

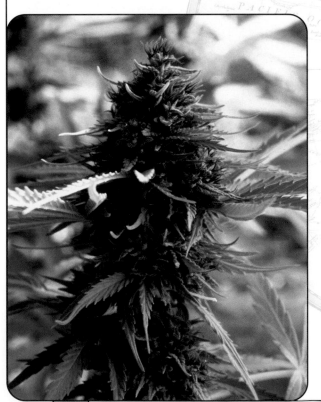

References to marijuana in the *Atharvaveda* texts of India are dated between 2000–1400 BC. Marijuana's presence in many areas of the world by mid-millennium is supported by the mention of cannabis and hemp in historical and literary documents of many countries. It is also one of the earliest plants to be cultivated. Within the family of cannabis, genetic differences in plants have combined with selection processes and environmental factors to result in some predictable characteristics based on the region of the world where that strain has been cultivated.

Globalization became relevant to marijuana long before its current attention in the press. Since the 1970s, the interchange of cannabis strains across national lines has accelerated. The popularization and success of indoor growing methods, and the development of breeding as a business mean that many strains of pot once particular to a specific region have migrated, or become international citizens. Some regions have lost original strains or have been hybridized through the inrush of other commercial varieties. Marijuana's migratory patterns around the world are a political story as much as they are a botanical one. Here, in brief, are some descriptions of marijuana's appearance in different regions of the world.

A plant in the Hindu Kush region, most likely marijuana's birthplace
photo credit: Mel Frank

India has tended to process plants for marijuana rather than hashish, making the lengthy history of selection and cultivation of special interest to many breeders.

The varieties of India tend to be tall plants with copious branching, especially toward the top of the plant. The buds, while fairly small, slim, and banana-shaped, tend to form at many sites on the plant, making for a desirable yield. Although hash production is not as prevalent, Indian varieties are impressively resinous. Taste and aroma are as fragrantly spicy as incense, and the high is notably psychoactive. Marijuana in India is typically referred to as ganja, which specifically means the flower tops. Other names used in India suggest the specific processing or product, and include *charas* (finger hash from flower tops), *bhang* (a chai-like marijuana beverage) and *kief* (glands shaken from leaves; unpressed hash). It is also associated with Shiva in Hindu legends, thus the use of this name for varieties by some breeders.

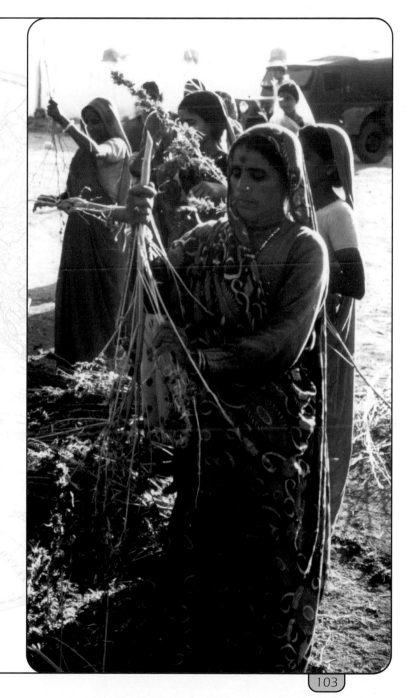

Women manicuring marijuana in India
photo credit: Ed Rosenthal

The island of **JAMAICA** lies in the heart of the Caribbean. Jamaica has a reputation for its acceptance of marijuana, which remains illegal despite attempts to change its legal status since 1999. It is widely tolerated within Jamaican society, and has common recreational and medicinal uses in addition to being considered a spiritual sacrament among Rastafarians. It is believed that marijuana was originally brought to Jamaica for spiritual use from India. Perhaps this is why the term *ganja* is used in both cultures, although Jamaica uses the term more generally. "Lamb's bread" is the name given to superior marijuana in Jamaica, and can usually only be found within the country.

Jamaicans also refer to cannabis as "Kali weed"–think killer weed, since Kali is the name of the Indian goddess of destruction.

In the heyday of the 1960s and 1970s, Jamaican varieties were commonplace in the world market. Around that time, Caribbean marijuana provided about one-fifth of the total cannabis consumed in the world. Now it accounts for less than one-twentieth. Increased pressure from the U.S. and competition from Mexico are in part responsible for the decline of Jamaican strains' international availability. This island's domestic marijuana has also been affected by the introduction of commercial Colombian and Mexican strains.

Traditional Jamaican varieties tend to be tall with a straight main branch and extensive side branching. The leaves are light green in color with serration along the edges. While they tend to be hardy, they prefer the long hot equatorial sunshine to more temperate zones, and may refuse to adapt to less favorable weather. Given the spiritual uses for which Jamaica is renowned, as well as the use of ganja to make repetitive manual labor easier to perform, many varieties show selection for a high that is alert, cerebral, and psychoactive, rather than strongly physical or sleepy in nature.

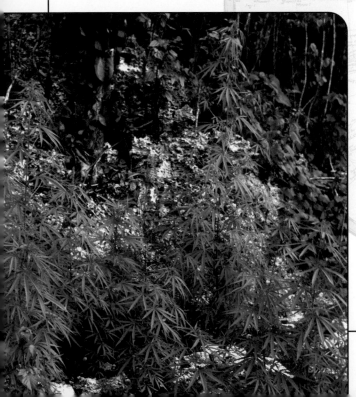

These outdoor plants show the straight growth patterns of native Jamaican ganja
photo credit: Ed Rosenthal

Located in east-central Africa, **MALAWI** is a small, landlocked country bordered to the east by Lake Malawi, and by Zambia and Mozambique to the west and southeast. The marijuana from this region has many lovely qualities. The plants tend to be medium in size with slender, drooping finger-like leaves of a deep green color spread widely along the stems, which makes manicuring simple.

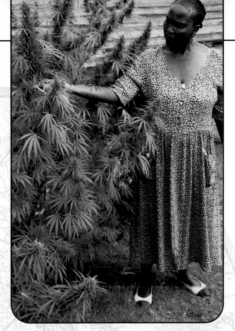

Here African Seed's Swazi Skunk grows outdoors in the environs of its homeland

While also equatorial like their Colombian and Jamaican cousins, Malawi varieties have shown more success in adapting to other latitudes and conditions. Malawi varieties form fairly large and loose buds, and tend to have a spicy flavor and a strong, mentally stimulating high.

Malawi marijuana is often wrapped in corn husks, termed "cobs." Cobs are used as a waterproof package, similar to a baggie. This allows cannabis to be transported by water, to cross borders, or traverse long distances. Because this practice is particular to Malawi, the term "Malawi Cob" may be used to refer to a bag of pot.

In **SOUTH AFRICA**, marijuana is referred to as dagga (the double g is pronounced with a guttural sound). South Africa first banned cannabis in 1911. Nevertheless, illegal marijuana farming is supposedly the third largest cash crop here. South Africa is mostly semiarid, with a subtropical area along the east coast that borders the warm Indian Ocean. The Kwazulu/Natal and Transkei regions both lie in the subtropical east coast, known for its lush greenness and rolling hills. Kwazulu/Natal is well known as the home of the large coastal city of Durban, from which Durban Poison derives its name. Directly south along the coast from Durban is the region of Transkei, which is considered the main dagga-producing region in South Africa. The neighboring country of **SWAZILAND**, which borders South Africa's northeast corner, is also well renowned for their high quality pot.

The marijuana of South Africa has a great reputation. The plants are primarily sativa, but finish flowering as early as September in northern latitudes. They resemble Southeast

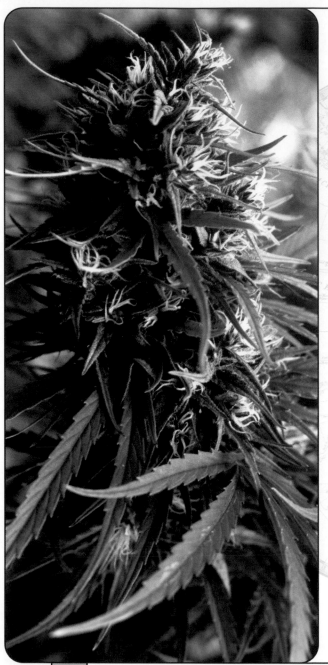

A classic Mexican variety
photo credit: Mel Frank

Asian varieties, with a fresh bouquet, a sweet anise-like taste when smoked, and an alert high. These plants are tall and elegant looking with long slender leaves and pale green buds. They often develop pink and purple tones at maturity.

• • • •

Cannabis from **MEXICO** derives from the mountainous regions. While it was once common to acquire premium varieties from Mexico, efforts by the U.S. to end the flow of drug traffic has lowered the quality of typical imported Mexican pot. In the 1960s and 1970s varieties from the states of Oaxaca, Guerrero, and Michoacan gained the most widespread popularity. Many Mexican strains in global circulation were named for their state of origin.

Plant appearance may vary from state to state, but most Mexican varieties are medium to tall in height with leaves varying in width, but typically dark green in color. Mexican varieties tend to have a fast to moderate growth cycle, outpacing most equatorial varieties. Many Mexican varieties also offer a buzz that is mentally stimulating and sativa-like in quality.

Mexican varieties started to decline in prevalence as Colombian strains flooded the market. In turn, Mexico began to export some green and brown commercial skunks and sinsemillas in great numbers into the western United States. Increased competition and intense efforts to eradicate marijuana traffic by the United States, including the use of Paraquat, resulted in a much diminished flow of marijuana from Mexico, with a lesser-quality commercial product now being commonly encountered by those outside of Mexico.

• • • •

NEPAL lies between India and Tibet, home to a magnificent part of the Himalayas, lying in the belt that is considered the ancient homelands of cannabis. While selection and cultivation occur here, unkempt marijuana plants can be encountered growing wild in the foothills.

Nepalese varieties tend to be leggy and only lightly branched, with long dense and very sensuous smelling buds at the top. Despite the number of untended or only loosely tended plants in Nepal, THC content remains good. They also produce impressive amounts of resin. The aroma of Nepalese strains may have been one of the defining varieties to describe the spicy hashish smell, sometimes referred to as "temple hash" because of its use in religious practice.

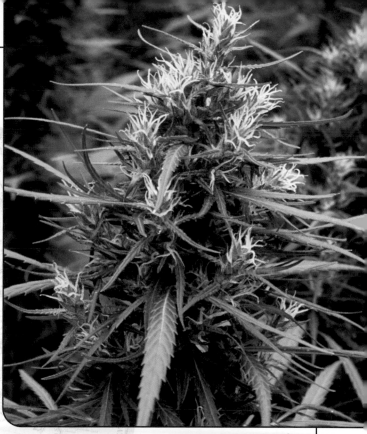

A young plant in Nepal
photo credit: Mel Frank

Closed to the outside world until the 1950s, Kathmandu became a hippie travel destination in the 1960s and 1970s, an exotic culture where marijuana was both cheap and legal. In part due to the publicity it received as a cannabis destination, marijuana was banned, and even though it is still available, legal public use of marijuana has been curbed, and foreign visitors are now subject to punishment for use.

RUSSIA is the home to a third, lesser known species of marijuana, Cannabis ruderalis. Distinct from both Cannabis indica and

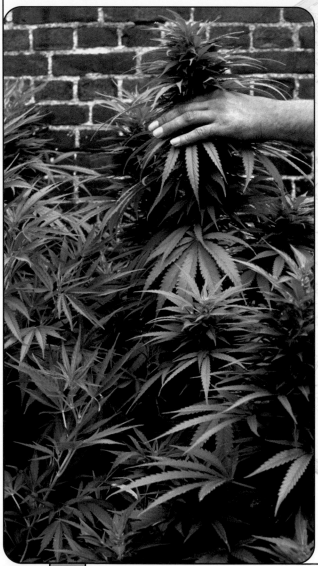

Cannabis sativa, C. ruderalis was encountered in Russia and named in 1924. Referred to as "weedy" cannabis, it is typically high in cannabidiol (CBD) one of the common cannabinoids, and low in THC content. Studies show that CBD content in marijuana often increases as the THC content decreases. Some cannabis strains have no CBD, such as those from Africa. Cannabis ruderalis may have remained below the radar for most marijuana enthusiasts because the smoke is nothing to brag about. The combination of a high CBD, low THC content results in a very sedative buzz that lacks psychoactive effects. CBD is non-psychoactive, but research in the last twenty years has shown that CBD has some remarkable medicinal properties, especially as an anti-inflammatory agent.

Russia's C. ruderalis plant is short, with a maximum height of about 1½ feet (50 centimeters). It grows as a single stem plant with wide squat leaves and smaller colas. The life cycle is short as is the flowering period. It also has the particular characteristic of autoflowering: that is, it flowers based on life cycle rather than the number of hours of light received per day. This trait tends to carry through hybridization, making it less desirable for this purpose.

This plant is an early ruderalis hybrid
photo credit: Ed Rosenthal

SOUTHEAST ASIA is made up of the countries of Cambodia, Laos, Thailand and Vietnam. While marijuana is cultivated throughout the Southeast Asian countries, especially in the northern and eastern tropical mountains and the eastern lowland regions, Thailand's pot may be the most well-known outside of this area. Thai stick is world famous, known as thick seedless buds, dried and wrapped carefully, usually in string. Typical Thai varieties tend to be very tall with large calyxes and long leaves composed of many leaflets. A strong main stem supports the extensive branching. The seeds are also very large. Thai strains are fruity in tone and tend toward the citrus in flavor.

Varieties from Thailand have a long growth cycle and are slow to flower. They also have a tendency toward hermaproditism, especially when changing to a more temperate climate. True strains can be a challenge even for an expert grower. However, hybrids created with hardy varieties that mature more quickly have increased chances of success. Thai strains, despite their difficulties have a very pleasant, powerful high that is worth the trouble. These plants have also reacted well to greenhouse growing set-ups in non-tropical locations.

As the demand for Thai marijuana increased in the world market, other cannabis strains were introduced and may have resulted in the hybridization of original Thai genetics. Regions of Southeast Asia have feral marijuana in patches that can be seen growing wild throughout the towns and tropical countryside.

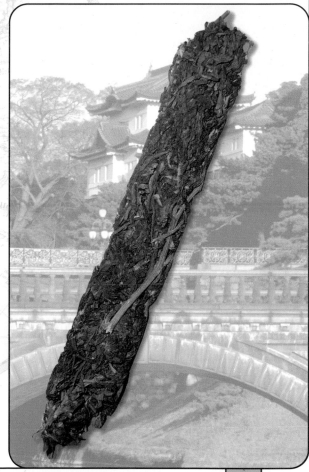

Thai Stick's name derives from its shape, which results from the drying and tying process
photo credit: Ed Rosenthal

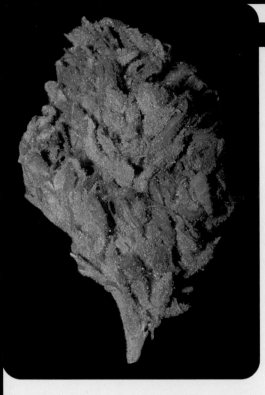

Nevil's Haze

 75/25

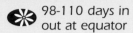 98-110 days in out at equator

 in preferred

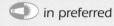 medium to low

 Haze x mystery indica

 psychedelic

pine, floral

Named for the breeder who began this hybrid, Nevil's Haze is a mostly Haze sativa that was crossed to be one-quarter indica. The Haze variety is renowned for being a tall gal, and Nevil's version follows it's genetically programmed desire to seek the sun by outgrowing its competitors.

Nevil's Haze leaves are very thin and long, with sparse buds and long internodes. This strain has a pine cone smell with a distinctively floral haze edge. The resin is abundant and the high is very potent and cerebral, encouraging a spiritual or philosophical disposition. With a THC content of 11 percent, Nevil's Haze can also induce a kick-in-the-pants, psychedelic type of buzz. CBD has been tested at 1.2 percent and CBN present at .1 percent.

Recommended as an indoor plant, this is a variety for those with the patience to wait the full 10 weeks required for a proper finish. Gardeners can skip the vegetative growth cycle and go straight to a 12/12 light schedule. This serves to control the height, and can also compensate somewhat for the long flowering time. Hydroponic methods are preferred indoors, but soil can also be workable. Forget growing this outdoors if you aren't within 20 degrees latitude of the equator. Nevil's Haze needs that long season of intense sun, and will be hard pressed to finish outside in most parts of the world. A real connoisseur plant, Nevil's Haze resists stressors well as long as tropics conditions are met.

Winner, *High Times* Cannabis Cup 1998

New Purple Power

 S

 56-63 days or mid-Oct out

 Purple Haze x Early Skunk

 clear/up

500–1000 g per plant

sour candy smell, tropical sweet flavor

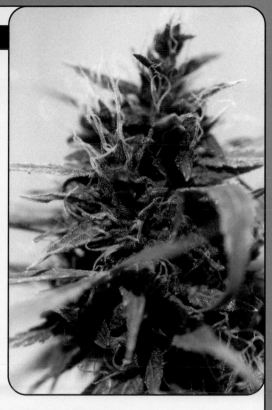

I n the late 1980s, the famous import purple strains were very popular to smoke but would not grow as well in the northern European regions. New Purple Power (NPP) was developed so the qualities of the yummy purple strains could be cultivated successfully in cold and wet climates.

Like all outdoor strains, New Purple Power appreciates lots of sun and warmth, but thrives even in the less reliable Dutch weather. The appearance is classic sativa, with long stems that are purple from the very start. The leaves have numerous thin fingers, and budding sites are plentiful.

A good producer, NPP's buds are darker purple if finished in a cooler environment. This plant can reach heights of over 6 feet (2 meters) in greenhouses and southern climates—in temperate climates New Purple Power averages around 5 feet (1.5 meters).

NPP has a mild but distinct sweet and sour smell, like a sour candy. The taste is tropical, and sweeter than the smell. NPP smokes mild and has little expansion. The buzz is clear and upbeat. Many heads like to toke NPP during the day, since the high leaves them happily buzzed, but still awake and functional.

Winner, *High Times* Cannabis Cup 1998

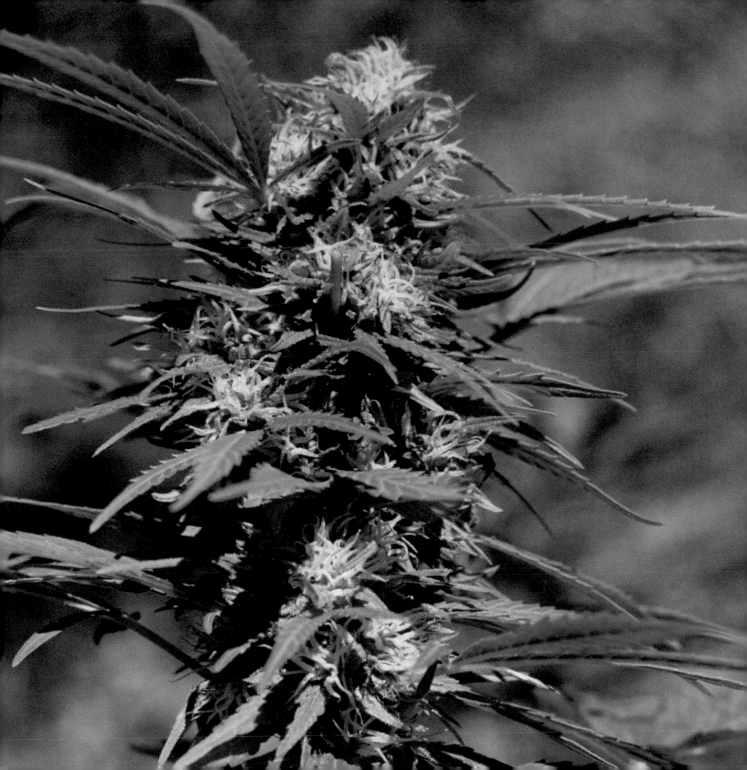

SI 75/25

 45-55 days in mid-Oct out

 400-500 g per dried, manicured plant out

SOG

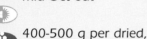 Oaxacan sativa x Afghani indica

 up

 earthy

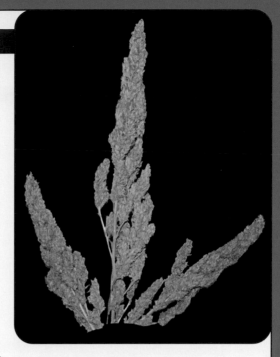

Some traveling stories lie behind this variety. In formulating Niagara, Dr. Greenthumb collected seeds from Oaxaca in Mexico and Jalalabad, which is east of Kabul in Afghanistan. The Oaxacan strain possessed sweet, heavy-yielding buds with hardly a leaf. The smoke was also wonderfully potent, but the finish was suitable to its Mexican homeland rather than the eastern coast of Canada. When combined with the Afghani strain that was accustomed to temperate latitudes, the resultant variety retained the lovely, clear and alert high and minimal foliage, but easily finished outdoors at 43 degrees latitude.

Named Niagara to conjure an association with its Canadian birthplace, this variety has been selectively bred over the decades for a shorter height and earlier finish. This is a dark green plant with dark colored buds and a full-bodied flavor reminiscent of the Canadian forests where it can happily dwell. Besides being a reliable outdoor plant, Niagara will grow in an indoor set-up using hydro or soil methods. The high flower-to-leaf ratio makes this a breeze to manicure upon finish.

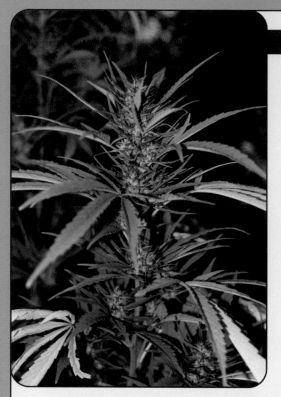

 50/50

 50-60 days

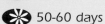 250-350 dried, manicured g per plant out

 Niagara x Shiva

 alert, giggly

 earthy, sweet

SOG

Niagara x Shiva was developed as a cross in order to capture the happy, silly effect of Sensi's Shiva in combination with Niagara's devastating potency. The resulting plant is a half and half indica/sativa mix that offers a more irreverent happy buzz and lighter taste than the Niagara while still proving easy to grow in the great outdoors of northern climates.

An average-sized plant, Niagara x Shiva will range between 4-6 feet (120-180 cm) outside and will stay around 2 feet (60 cm) in an indoor grow. This is a wonderfully versatile hybrid that will thrive by any method as long as the generally recommended conditions are met. As it matures, Niagara x Shiva often gets purple pistils but keeps the leaf count to a minimum, maintaining the easy manicuring trait of its Niagara parent.

Not as sweet as its Amsterdam sweet Shiva parent, this variety has a well-rounded, down-home earthy flavor with a hint of the woods. The buzz is a special mixture of high, with potent and mood shifting effects, offering a euphoric giggly sensation that is great for summer days, music festivals or a comedy movie marathon.

Dr. Greenthumb's Cannabis Travels:

"In 1968, I took my first trip in search of good and abundant smoke. At that time, I'd been smoking for a year or two and I'd heard about potent cannabis in Mexico, so it seemed natural to go to the source. After all, the price of a pound in Canada had skyrocketed from $80 to $250 almost overnight. Mexico was great! The pot was cheap, not to mention potent and abundant. My traveling buddy and I bought green trash bags full of untrimmed colas for under $100 U.S. at Pie de la Quetsta, near Acapulco, plus a few shoeboxes' full at Oaxaca . . . life was good!

When I returned to Canada, I tried to grow out some of the seeds I'd acquired, but of course nature and bad luck played their hands. The Oaxacan was stolen that October even though it was nowhere near finishing.

The following year, a friend and I decided to go on a 4-month tour of India, Nepal, Pakistan and Afghanistan. The hash was outstanding. Most notable were dark, dark black from Bombay; Nepalese Fingers and Temple Balls from around Nepalgange; Kashmiri resin from Srinigar; and from Afghanistan, Kanhari Moon Discs and Jalalabad Spaghetti Sticks. Even the raw chunks of resin commercially available were excellent smoke.

It was pure luck that I brought any seeds back to Canada. It had never occurred to me to collect seeds until one day we bought some super-potent resin chunks in Jalalabad and were surprised that they contained the odd seed. The seeds were notable because they were so very large—we referred to them as ping pong balls. I saved them, seven in all, and took them back to Canada. This was the seed that was crossed with the Oaxacan to produce Niagara.

I've done a lot of traveling over the years, but always to cannabis-producing countries. Since the formation of Greenthumb Seeds in 1995, some travel has been in order to search for pure gene stock for breeding purposes. But both before and since forming my company, I have made it a point to only travel where cannabis is produced, if not to collect seeds, then to show my support, and of course, to sample and enjoy."

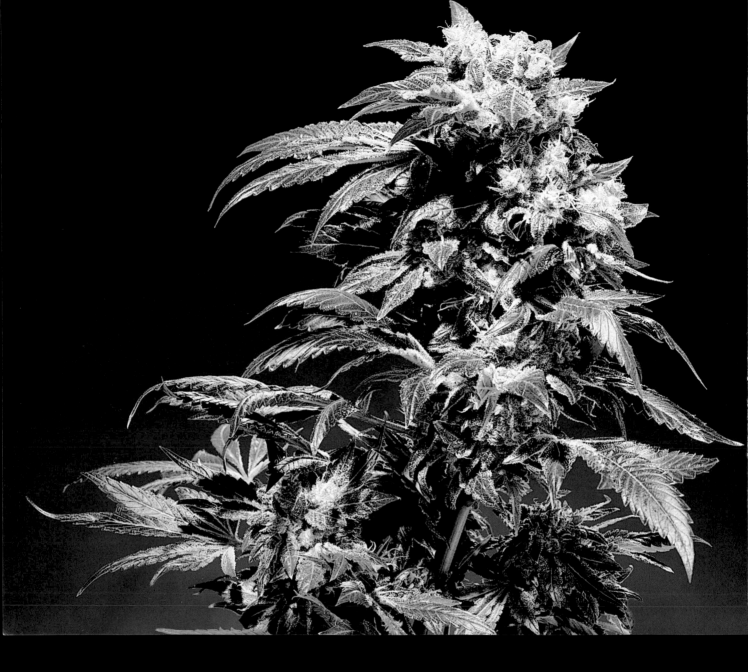

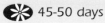

Northern Lights

 I

 45-50 days

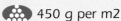 450 g per m2

 Northern Lights 5
x Northern Lights 2

 narcotic, body high

sweet, pungent, spicy

SOG

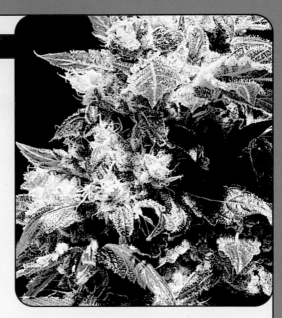

The Northern Lights (NL) is one of the most potent and famous indica varieties. Even though there are a lot of copies circulating around with variations on the name, there are only 3 pure types from the original development of Northern Lights, which Sensi was lucky to acquire.

Historically, the NL 1, a longer, more stretchy type with a fresh scent and good bud formation, was the basis of the NL cross that was sold as Sensi's Northern Lights. Currently, the NL 5 has taken over the most important role in the cross. Because NL 5 adds potency and reduces flowering time, but is not dominant in taste and smell, it also plays a starring role in the overall breeding plan at the Cannabis Castle. It has functioned as a test case for many crosses. The f1 generation is very predictable, giving uniform results and passing uniformity on to the hybrids it parents. The NL 2 contributes to the overall vigor of the plant and strength of the high, also lending its spider mite resistance to the cross.

Highly adapted to indoor growing, Northern Lights is a satisfying yielder that can finish in just over 6 weeks. The best results are obtained from hydro culture gardens. Small sea of green plants or bigger indoor plants will both do well, but remember that yield is directly related to the amount of light and space.

A petite plant averaging between 3½-5 feet (110-150 cm), NL has dense, resin-rich flowers and wide-fingered indica leaves. The aroma is pungently sweet and the taste is a flavorful mixture of sweet and spicy. The high is a potent physical experience that feels comfortably lazy and relaxing.

Northern Light's fame extends to the harvest festivals where it claimed the overall *High Times* Cannabis Cup win in 1990, and the Cup's award for the pure Indica category in 1988-89.

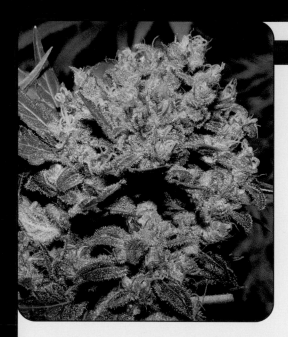

Northern Lights x Bubble Gum

 I

 49-60 days

 90-120 g per plant in; up to 1 lb. per plant out

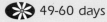 Northern Lights x Bubble Gum

lethargic

bubble gum

Northern Lights x Bubble Gum (NL x BG) is 50 percent of each parent and 100 percent indica. It has retained the stability and hardiness of the Northern Lights strains, and inherited the sweet smell of Bazooka Joe responsible for parent Bubble Gum's name.

Plants are medium-sized with

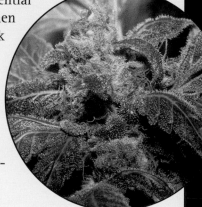

tight, small nuggets that appear at multiple sites to give a yield potential between 90-120 g per plant indoors, and up to a pound per plant when grown to a fully-branched plant under the sun. NL x BG grows a thick collection of hairs that turn amber as the buds mature. Flowering is rapid, with a finishing time between 7–9 weeks. This plant responds well to the photoperiod of the Northern hemisphere, making it a good guerilla garden variety in many temperate climates.

Northern Lights x Bubble Gum produces a heavy, lethargic body stone that is made for sweet dreams. Although it is good for sleeping, it can also result in a relaxed but thoughtful high. Dr. Atomic recommends this variety for all maladies.

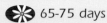
Northern Lights-Haze

 65-75 days

 Northern Lights 5 x Haze

 up, psychedelic

fresh/peppery

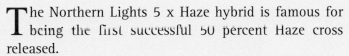 380 g per m2

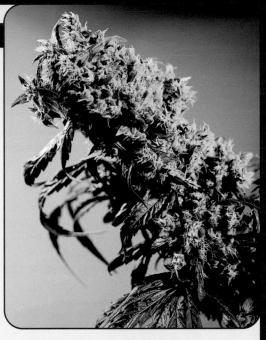

The Northern Lights 5 x Haze hybrid is famous for being the first successful 50 percent Haze cross released.

The Haze is a long (up to 6 months) flowering sativa from the U.S. Very popular in the 1970s, it became nearly extinct in the late 1980s because growers were switching to easier, higher-yielding varieties. Breeders at the Cannabis Castle crossed Haze genetics with the uniform and quick-finishing NL 5 indica to make a lush producer with a refreshing high.

Due to the radically sativa nature of the Haze, this cross stretches a lot and takes a longer flowering period to finish than most common cannabis hybrids. This stretchy quality also allows cuttings to enter flowering as soon as they are rooted. Some growers even start the seeds under a 12-hour light regimen with success. This early entry into flowering phase allows NL-Haze to finish in a similar amount of time as conventional, indica-heavy crosses that need more vegetative time. The growth tendencies of the NL-Haze are enhanced when grown as larger plants and diminished in a sea of green method.

Don't be tempted to harvest too early. Long flowering crosses can create some nail-biting for the grower, but tenacity and some experience pay off with buds of superb quality. NL-Haze delivers fresh, spicy sativa-type buds that have a clean, peppery taste. An immediate, cerebral high, this pot has sometimes been referred to as "speed weed" in Holland. Overall NL-Haze is a friendly high with a trippy edge that adds some extra zing to any day.

Winner, *High Times* Cannabis Cup overall 1994

Winner, *High Times* Cannabis Cup mostly sativa category 1990 and 1994

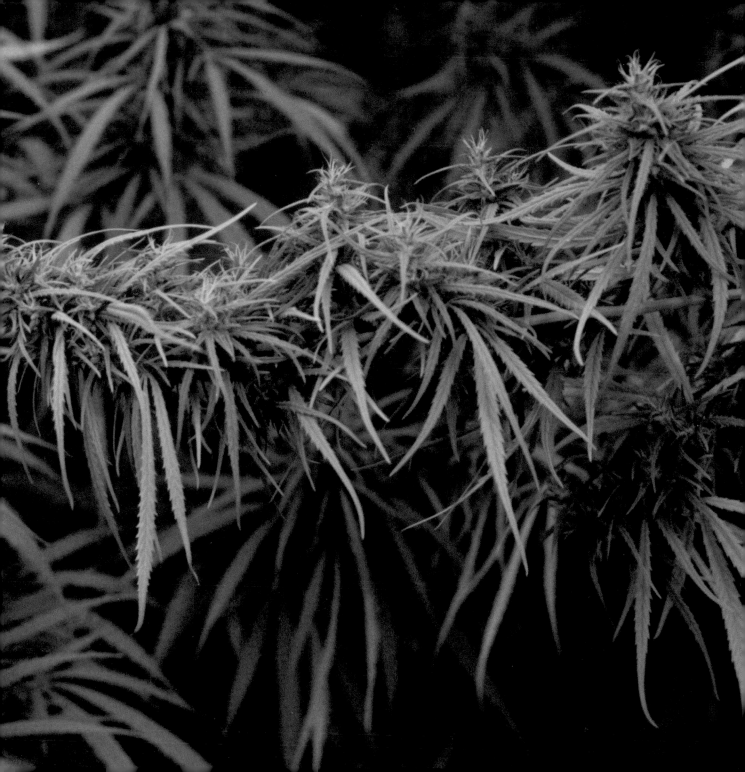

Old Mother Sativa

 S

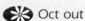 Oct out

 up to 5 lbs per plant

 sativa

 smooth, mellow

acrid/peppery

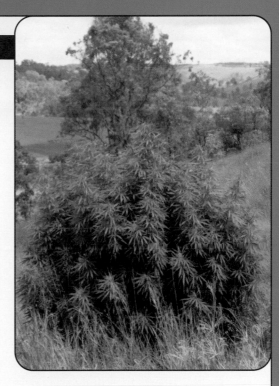

Kog has been growing Old Mother Sativa in Australia for the past 18 years. It is a very hardy plant, able to withstand severe drought and spring back when water is provided by the grower or mother nature. It also shows resistance to frost in the flowering phase. Selectively bred to be a humongous outdoor plant, Old Mother Sativa is well acclimatized to the Australian climate, at 30 degrees latitude S and low elevation.

Suspected to have Southeast Asian roots, this plant was popular among hippies of Australia in the heyday, especially around the Hunter Valley region where it thrived in the 1960s. Old Mother Sativa has a long growing season, and gives best results under full sun, planted in well-drained soil. The root system for this plant tends to be wide and shallow rather than deep, making hilltops and sandy soils along riverbanks super locations for planting. She can reach heights of 15 feet if given a long growing season over Australia's summer. In a short season, over winter, with less sunshine and warmth, she may remain at a foot tall and produce only about an ounce per plant.

In the wrong environment, or the hands of the inexperienced, this strain can produce a disappointing yield but allowed to grow to her mega-proportions, Old Mother can deliver a primeval harvest of up to 5 pounds. The smoke from this plant is delicious, mellow, and fun, perfect for a sweet silly time with friends. The clarity of this pure sativa will not leave you dozing off or locked to the couch. This plant is easy to clone and may develop purple coloring in cooler growing conditions.

Cannabis Across Canada
■ Dana Larsen

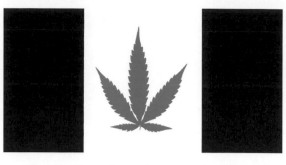

The marijuana activism scene in Canada experienced a rebirth in the early 1990s, when activists began opening "hemp stores" that openly defied the ban on paraphernalia and pro-pot literature and magazines.

One of the first such stores was Hemp Nation, in London Ontario, owned by Chris Clay. In 1994, Marc Emery opened a store called Hemp BC in Vancouver, also violating Canada's prohibition. The Hemp BC store was a hive of sales and activity, and served as the central focus of pot activism in BC for the next few years. Profits from Hemp BC funded activist projects, rallies and a newsletter that eventually grew into *Cannabis Culture* magazine. After meeting Sensi Seeds founder Ben Dronkers at the *High Times* Cannabis Cup, Emery was inspired to add a small selection of marijuana seeds. The seeds proved popular, and quickly became the financial backbone of the enterprise.

By 1995 the proliferation of hemp stores across Canada faced increasing legal pressure. Chris Clay was arrested and charged for selling some cannabis cuttings and seeds from his shop in May of that year. Thus began one of many legal challenges to the constitutionality of Canada's ban on marijuana. In December 1995, Ken Venema's hemp store, Kaiyun, was raided in Ontario. Emery's Hemp BC operation was raided in January 1996, exactly one month after Emery and his store were profiled on the front page of the *Wall Street Journal*.

During these raids, the police would empty out the store, taking out every single bong, pipe and pot seed on the premises. Sometimes they wouldn't even press charges for

Marc Emery (center) speaks at a rally in Vancouver, BC
photo credit: Ed Rosenthal

the seized paraphernalia, forcing the financial-ly devastated store owner out of business without the need for a trial.

Hemp BC reopened in 1997, expanding to include the Cannabis Cafe, the Little Grow Store, and the Hemp BC Legal Assistance Centre, only to be raided again, almost two years after the first, in December 1997. The raid was followed by a regular series of raids during 1998, so that Hemp BC and the Cannabis Cafe were shut down entirely.

There is now no overt over-the-counter outlets for marijuana seeds in Vancouver. There are some reputable places where seeds can be acquired, but most of the seed business takes place through mail-order only.

In 2001, Vancouver has a number of underground clubs where marijuana can be bought for a good price. A catering business called Stranjahs advertises that they will provide ganjalicious goodies for private parties. A few cafes allow patrons to smoke pot, but don't sell pot or tolerate any dealing on the premises.

Meanwhile, a number of "constitutional challenges" to marijuana prohibition are working

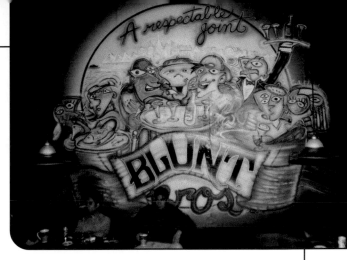

Mural in Vancouver's pot-friendly Blunt Bros. coffeeshop. photo credit: Ed Rosenthal

their way through the Canadian court system. Most of these challenges are being fought in court by dedicated lawyers John Conroy and Alan Young, and include both Terry Parker's and Jim Wakeford's challenges for medical use.

In 1987, epileptic Terry Parker was charged with possession of marijuana, but the judge accepted Parker's plea of "medical necessity" and acquitted him of possession charges, thus making him Canada's first semi-legal marijuana user. Despite this, Parker's apartment was raided by Toronto police nine years later in July 1996. They found 71 plants, and charged him with possession, cultivation and trafficking.

The Ontario Court of Justice again accepted Parker's defense in December 1997, and found him not guilty of possession and cultivation of marijuana, by reason of medical necessity. He was found guilty of trafficking after admitting he had given buds to other sick friends. The judge even ruled that Parker's pot plants should be returned, although the police failed to do so. The decision made headlines across Canada.

The feds appealed the decision to the Ontario Court of Appeal, taking the case to Ontario's highest court. In July 2000, the judge ruled that Canada's law against marijuana was unconstitutional, and granted Terry Parker the right to use medicinal marijuana. The judge also ruled that Parliament had one year to rewrite Canada's marijuana laws to accommodate med-pot usage, or else the pot-prohibition law would be completely erased from the Criminal Code.

Meanwhile, Ontario AIDS patient Jim Wakeford was fighting a court battle which ultimately forced Canada's government to grant him the nation's first "Section 56 exemption" to the ban on pot. Section 56 of Canada's Controlled Drugs and Substances Act allows the Minister of Health to grant individual exemptions to aspects of the drug laws, for scientific or medical purposes.

A pro-legalization rally in Vancouver, BC
photo credit: Ed Rosenthal

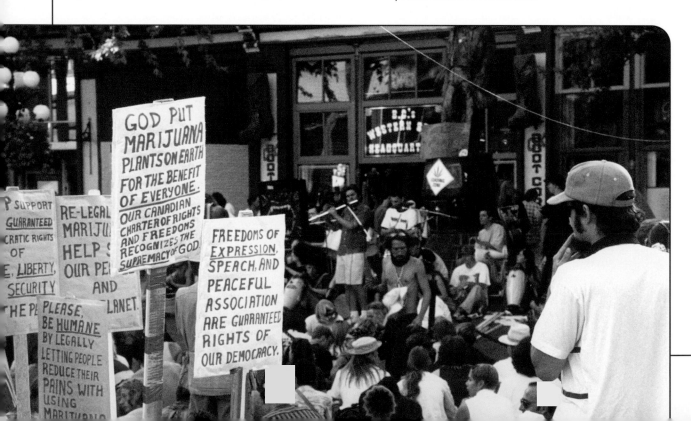

Wakeford received his exemption in May 1999, and by early 2001 over 200 other Canadians had also received exemptions for med-pot use. The process remains very slow and bureaucratically complex. Exemptees are not provided with pot or allowed to buy it from others. They must grow their own marijuana, but have no legal access to seeds or clones. They are also strictly limited to cultivating a small number of plants, and face police inspections and possible arrest if they violate any of the guidelines.

Many medical marijuana users buy their pot from an ever-increasing number of cannabis compassion clubs across Canada, which supply marijuana to those with a medical need. The largest of these is the BC Compassion Club, which sells medical pot to over 1500 clients from their clinic in downtown Vancouver. The club was founded in 1997 and has never suffered a police raid, although other Canadian clubs have.

Canada's Liberal government is slowly moving toward access to marijuana for medical purposes. New regulations which came into force July 31,

2001, allow patients to designate a caregiver who can grow marijuana for them, and expand the range of illnesses for which marijuana can be used. Although many patients and doctors still have serious complaints

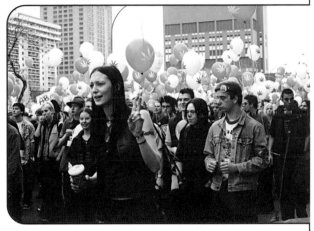

Montreal marchers fill the streets in support of pot legalization. photo credit: Spanner McNeil

about the complexity and invasiveness of the regulations, no one can deny that Canada's prohibition against marijuana, and medical marijuana in particular, is fracturing in the face of increasing public pressure and court decisions.

Canada's marijuana liberation activists have also moved to directly challenge the status quo in the political arena. In 1997 the Province of Quebec saw the formation of

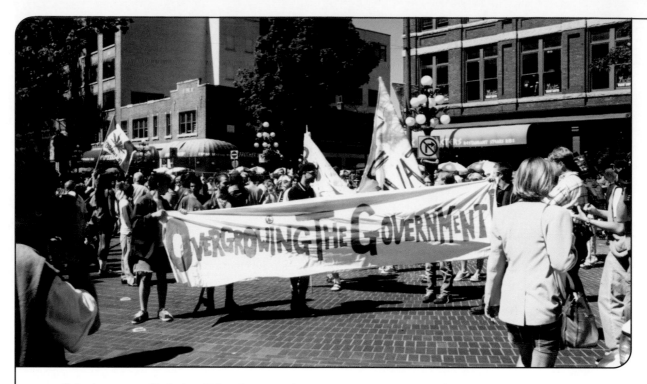

a political party called the "Bloc Pot," a play on the name of Quebec's sovereigntist political party, the Bloc Quebecois. The Bloc Pot ran in Quebec's 1998 provincial elections and gathered 1.25 percent of the vote.

In 2000, Bloc Pot founder and leader Marc-Boris St-Maurice traveled across Canada working with local activists to create a national political party devoted to cannabis liberation. The Canada Marijuana Party was born, with candidates all across the country running in Canada's November 2000 federal election. Most candidates averaged between 2-3 percent of the popular vote, and in some ridings beat out the more established Green, Alliance and NDP candidates.

In January 2001, activists in BC got together and formed the BC Marijuana Party, running in BC's May election. Marc Emery became BC party president, financing the campaign and coordinating candidates, while Party Leader Brian Taylor, past mayor of Grand Forks, BC, traveled the province in the "Canna-Bus" campaigning for local candidates. The BC Marijuana Party has received a special mention in the BC election archives for being the first party in the province's history to run a full slate of 79 candidates in their very first election. The party received about 53,000 votes, 3.5 percent of the popular vote.

Nova Scotia activists have already registered the Nova Scotia Marijuana Party, and other Canadian provinces are working toward forming their own local marijuana parties, so that within a few years there should be a Marijuana Party candidate of some kind running in every single election—federal, provincial or municipal—everywhere in Canada.

Many Canadians hope that continuing activism,

protest, and legal challenges will finally break the back of prohibition in Canada, giving all Canadians access to the benefits of the world's most amazing plant.

Dana Larsen has served as editor of *Cannabis Culture* magazine since its inception in 1994. He has written hundreds of articles and essays on cannabis and drug policy, history and related issues. Dana is also a founding member of the BC and Canadian Marijuana Parties, and is the author of the *Pot Puzzle Fun Book*. *Cannabis Culture* can be accessed online at www.cannabisculture.com.

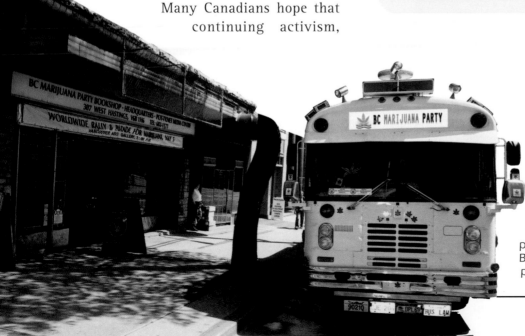

Former President Reagan's tour bus has found a new home with the BC Marijuana Party as the "Canna-Bus," parked here outside of the BC Party headquarters
photo credit: Ed Rosenthal

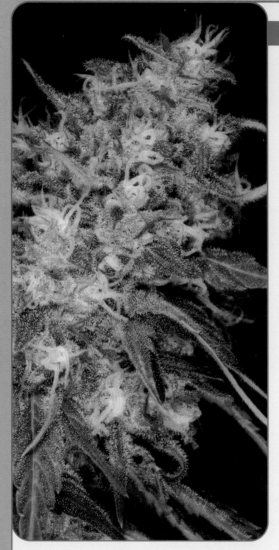

Original Misty

 I

 Misty x Misty

 49-63 days

 body stone

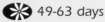

 sweet

600 g per m2

SOG

The Original Misty earns her name from the mist of THC glands that grace her buds and leaves like a dewy carpet. This plant is well-adapted to indoor techniques, producing a consistently high yield that averages a gram of bud per watt of light, even for beginning gardeners. Hydroponic or soil methods are both suitable for this all-indica original. While not suitable for the Dutch climate, Original Misty may find success in the great outdoors if grown in arid Mediterranean-type climates.

This variety delivers fat buds with a gourmet taste and sweet aroma. Original Misty has an enviable degree of uniformity in growth patterns, making her very happily suited to a sea of green planting method, where plants can be placed closely, improving the yield per square meter. Given her genetic tendency toward bushiness, this plant will also make a good larger plant with multiple branches.

Original Misty offers a pacifying high. Smoke this stoney weed when you don't plan on leaving the couch for much more than a trip to the kitchen for snacks. This is also great weed for the hash fan or ganja chef, since the kief will be plentiful and process well into butter or other cooking products.

Pot of Gold

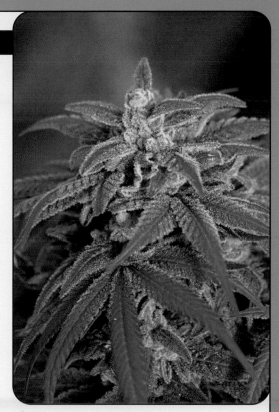

 I

 56-70 days in Oct out

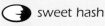 up to 600 g per m2 with 600 wpm

 Skunk #1 (m) x Hindu Kush (f)

 couch lock

 sweet hash

SOG

Pot of Gold is a stable hybrid. The Hindu Kush mother is a long-maintained pure strain from the mountains of Afghanistan. The Skunk#1 father is a Mexican/Colombian/pure Afghani cross. Both parents of this plant came from California to Holland in 1985 with a legendary cannabis enthusiast and breeder.

Pot of Gold matures into a medium to dark green plant with dense bud formations and only a few leaves that are between a sativa and indica shape. She will reach a medium height and form a thick canopy. Trimming the lower branches will concentrate the buds closer to the light, increasing total yield. With its strongly Afghan heritage, the buds and leaves are extremely resinous, crying out to be raw material for hashish. Flying Dutchmen advises gardeners to grow fully organically on soil, the only method they use. Keep the air flowing and the humidity down. Like all densely-flowered heavy producers, this exceptionally delicious plant needs a watchful eye to keep mold attacks at bay.

Pot of Gold will reward a gardener's extra vigilance with a mesmerizing and intense high, a smell like the sweetest hashish, and a taste that is hashy with some fruit.

Honorable Mention, *High Times* Cannabis Cup 1998

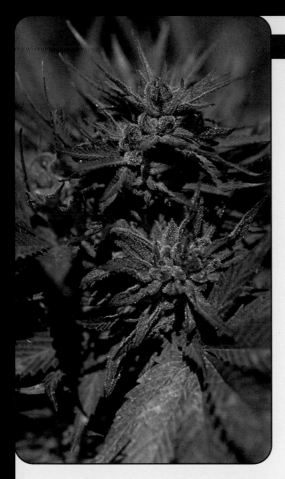

The Pure Skunk #1

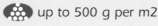

 75/25

 56 days in; Oct out

 up to 500 g per m2

 Mexican Colombian (f) x Afghani (m)

 cerebral

sweet

S kunk #1 seeds are the direct and unadulterated descendants of the stable hybrid Skunk #1 that was created in California in the late 1970s and brought to Holland in 1985. Despite the name, this variety has none of the acrid smell usually associated with pure Afghani strains. "The Pure" has a sweet smell and a full, satisfying taste.

Skunk #1 is a 75 percent sativa with a modified sativa appearance—it stays shorter than most sativas with leaves that are few and large, and short internodes. The big flowers range in color from lime green to gold at harvest. Although the buds are dense, they allow enough airflow to avoid mold problems. Resistance to molds makes The Pure a perfect variety for greenhouse cultivation where high-quality, heavy dense buds and uniformity are essential. The Afghani parent speeds up the finishing time to 8 weeks indoors.

Flying Dutchmen regularly yields 500 grams per square meter when growing this variety in a greenhouse in soil. They recommend using all-organic medium and fertilizer for the highest quality results. This strain offers all the flavor and the clear, cerebral effects of a sativa with the quick maturation of an indica. The Pure Skunk #1 was awarded the very first *High Times* Cannabis Cup in 1987.

Flying Dutchmen on the Skunk #1

Back in the 1960s, the scene in Holland was more hashish than pot, as the available grass was mostly mediocre imported stuff. By the mid-1970s, a small number of Dutch enthusiasts started growing at home. The first strains were large plants with small buds of average taste and high, but a few seeds eventually made it over from Afghanistan. Then this weird character from the States showed up with some new varieties: pure breeding strains from Colombia, Afghanistan and South Africa. More importantly, he brought over a few crosses he had made himself, including the Skunk #1, earning him the nickname, "The Skunk Man."

The Skunk #1 was a Colombian/Mexican/ Afghani cross. Flying Dutchmen breeder, Eddy, was one of the main enthusiasts in the growing scene at the time, and while initially skeptical about the Skunk Man's claims, he decided to grow out this guy's seeds and let the results speak for themselves. Eddy used the greenhouse method of simulated day and night cycles that predated the current indoor growing revolution. In 1984, the first crop was grown out and the results were so astounding, Eddy knew he'd found the future of Dutch weed, and never looked back.

Eddy says that the Skunk #1 was the first true stabilized hybrid in Holland's marijuana world, changing the trajectory of cannabis in the Netherlands. According to him, the initial selection was more fundamental than the breeding in making the Skunk #1 what it is. The combination of Afghani and sativa genetics brought together the best of both worlds.

The one conundrum remains this variety's widely known name—contrary to expectation, the taste is delicate, more floral than anything, and completely lacking the pungent tones that the word "skunk" evokes. Flying Dutchmen has employed the pure strains of the Skunk Man in many varieties, using other strains he introduced as mother plants and a hybridized Skunk #1 as the father. The original Skunk #1 line is also made available as "The Pure," in appreciation of the Skunk Man's contribution to the evolution of breeding.

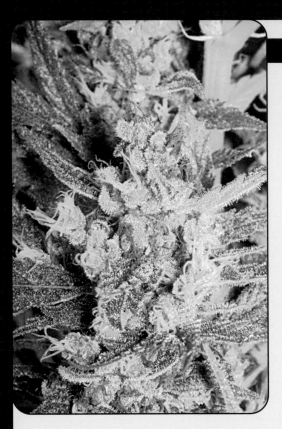

The Real McCoy

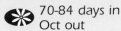

 60/40

 70-84 days in Oct out

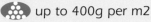 up to 400g per m2

Hawaiian (f) x Skunk #1 (m)

cerebral

sweet, spicy

The Real McCoy weds a Hawaiian mother with the Skunk #1 male. This plant makes her mostly sativa heritage obvious in her growth habits, getting tall and light green in tone, with long slender leaves and moderately tight buds. Real McCoy stretches a bit in flowering, and develops side branches that can grow quite long. Gardeners can use pruning or bending and staking techniques to make this trait an advantage.

The flowering phase takes a minimum of 10 weeks, making the Real McCoy a better choice for indoors or greenhouse cultivation. Flying Dutchmen prefers growing in a completely organic garden using soil, but also finds this variety to be happy as a greenhouse plant because the buds are loose enough to resist mold but dense enough to give moderate yields. Outdoor gardens in Holland have finished in October.

The Real McCoy cures to a citrus smell with no hint of indica's acrid trait. The taste is sweet and spicy at the same time, and produces a happy cerebral buzz that enhances any daytime activities, whether active or reflective in nature. At the 1999 *High Times* Cannabis Cup, The Real McCoy received a special mention from the celebrity judges.

Reclining Buddha

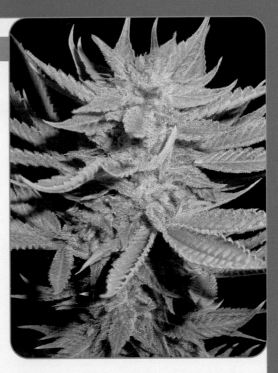

 I

❋ 63 days

 15-20 g per plant in 1 gal. pot

 Super Skunk x
Big Skunk Korean x
Holland's Hope

🐝 cerebral, creative

👅 sweet

SOG

Reclining Buddha is a 3-way hybrid that combines the genetics of Holland's Hope with Super Skunk and Big Skunk Korean. Circulating in the Netherlands during the 1980s, Holland's Hope is a mold-resistant strain with a very close nodal structure whose name can be attributed to her success in outdoor grows, even in Holland's wettest season. Reclining Buddha has held this characteristic, and combined it with the enjoyable smell and yields of its other two parents. Previously named Soma Skunk V, the new, enlightened name came out of a philosophical session prompted under her influence.

A fairly short plant, Reclining Buddha must remain in vegetative phase for a considerable amount of time to become a big plant. She also will not make a lot of side branches, and the ones that she does make tend to be smaller, a combination that predisposes this variety to do well with minimal effort in a sea of green set-up. Reclining Buddha's buds are tight and narrow, allowing moisture to escape easier than short, thicker bud formations. Try this one outdoors even in humid locations for a covert plant that delivers high-quality yield.

Buddha buds form many dark auburn hairs early. When everything around it still has white hairs, Reclining Buddha's hairs have turned a color that tempts you to harvest, but exercise patience. Reclining Buddha needs a full 9 weeks to reach maturity, and the high just gets better with the wait.

This medicinal quality cannabis has the taste of a sweet cherry candy and an uplifting creative high that is lucid and mentally stimulating.

3rd place, *High Times* Cannabis Cup, best indica 1999

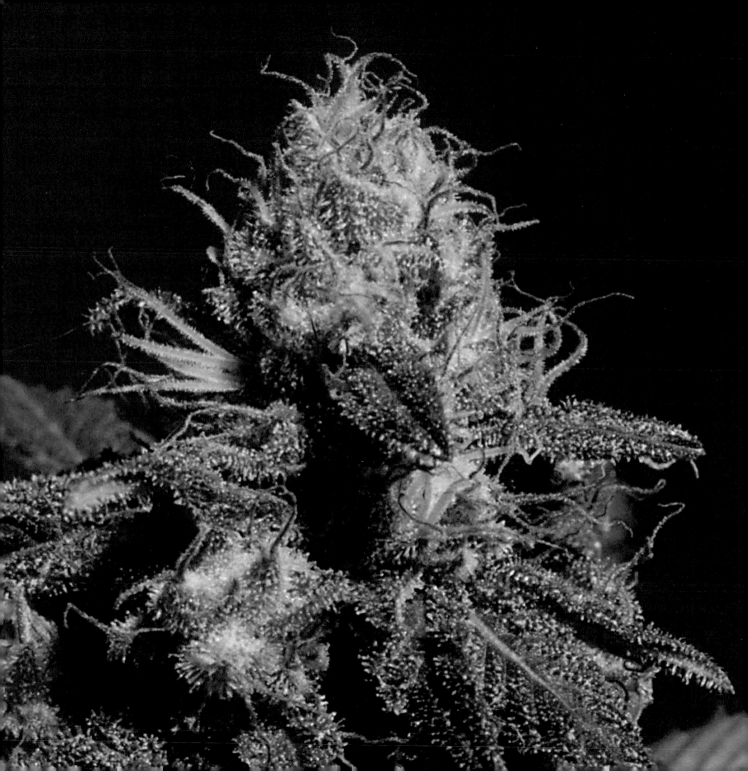

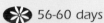

Romulan

 I

 56-60 days

 California strain x White Rhino backcrossed

 heavy

up to 1 oz per plant
2 gal. pot in
1/2 lb per plant out

dry, pungent, spicy

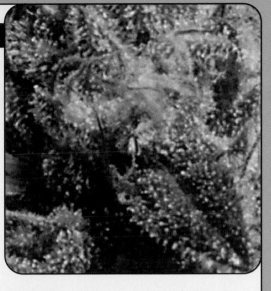

Federation purchased Romulan as a complete strain in 1996 in an attempt to rescue it from extinction. In the 1970s, this variety was brought from California to British Columbia by a Vietnam veteran, where it was grown on Vancouver Island. This variety was nicknamed Romulan after people joked that the high could "dent your head," producing ridges like those of Star Trek's warrior-like race with the same name.

Federation acquired Romulan in the form of clones, so she was entirely female. After crossing it with a Cannabis Cup prizewinner, a White Rhino male, breeders at Federation backcrossed 11 times to stabilize the variety at a 97 percent pure Romulan hybrid. Selections at each backcross favored the biggest, most robust plants over the fastest, although the finishing time remains around a very acceptable 8 weeks. Romulan seeds are now homogeneous and have an improved robustness and yield as a result.

This purple-stemmed plant branches extensively and is less appropriate for a sea of green garden than a set-up which takes advantage of the multiple branching and budding sites. A completely indica plant, Romulan is short and bushy with dark green leaves and thick buds. While still a moderate producer, Romulan has not lost its head-denting capabilities, and claims the title of Federation's most potent strain. Outdoors, this plant will yield about a half-pound of tight nuggets per fully grown plant. Drier climates are more favorable since the buds, being both thick and dense, have some susceptibility to mold.

Romulan is alien pot with potent effects. Couch lock is likely and concentration may be difficult to maintain. Medically, this weed has shown excellent results for chronic pain. In addition to its ongoing popularity in BC, Romulan has developed a devoted fan base in Texas.

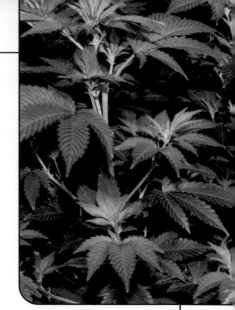

Tony of Sagarmatha on stabilizing strains:

"Every time you do in-line breeding, there's a possibility of something really noticeably changing. Part of it is knowing your plants. It also helps if you're lucky enough to have a lot of individuals to choose from. If you have a selection, the hard part is the males, so what you'll have to do is find all your females and then take 4 or 5 males that you think are going to be vigorous and show signs of flowering the fastest. You take those males and cross them against clones from the females. You won't know which females are nice until the very end of the day, because what may be a vigorous grower during the first or middle part of the thing may not be a good finisher, or vice versa. You have to make a lot of clones during this process. You may not have enough room to take 20 clones off of one variety, so you'll take 5 and when you figure out which ones you want, you have to grow those out, and make enough copies to fulfill your seed needs. It can be a lot of work, keeping all the records straight, with everything tagged and numbered. It's a real drag sometimes when you're working on a project and you may be using some pollen stored from the males you had collected, and it didn't

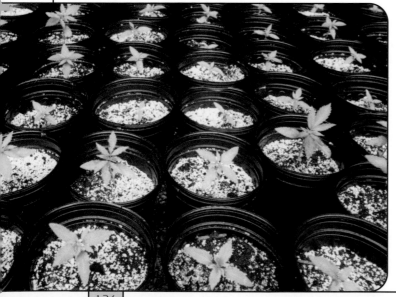

work out right, or for whatever reason the seeds just didn't take. You've got to start again and there goes another 6 months. It takes a lot of work to keep a whole menu of seeds fresh and up-to-date. We use multiple methods for stability in addition to in-line breeding, and we rotate crops every 2 to $2\frac{1}{2}$ years. Seeds have a maximum shelf life of 4-5 years for optimal germination rates. So if someone ordered seeds at the end of a seeds cycle, they would still have around 3 years before germination rates drop. The germination rate in the first 4-5 years should be about 90 percent. Every year after that, it decreases about 10 percent per year."

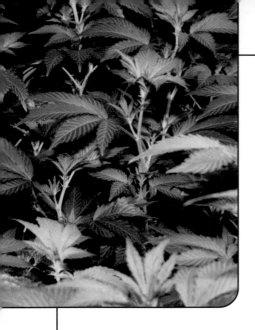

Breeder Shantibaba of Mr. Nice Seed Bank on stabilizing:

"It takes 5 generations to make a stable breed. Obviously this takes 5 seasons outdoors, but since all my breeding is done inside, I can do 5 generations in about a year and a half, allowing for a few muck-ups.

If you begin with a known breed, say a 100 percent pure sativa, that you would like to stabilize, you find the best female and the best male, and cross them. This is the f1 generation. Select the best male from the f1 and the best female and cross them to arrive at f2. The best female from f2 should be crossed to the original father you began with to produce the f3. Select the best male from the f3 and cross it back with the original mother. You are now at f4, which should be a stable breed producing uniform results. To test that the breeding was all true, the f4s are interbred among themselves, and the seeds are grown out to test for uniformity. Another way of doing it is to begin with the mother and father, interbreed 3 or 4 times, then cross the selected females to the original papa male to test the seed for uniformity."

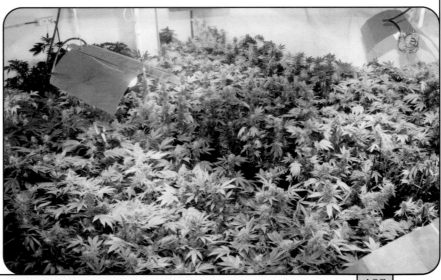

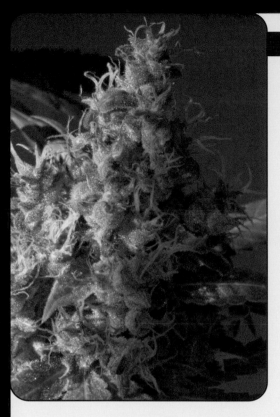

SAGE

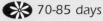 70-85 days

 Big Sur Holy x Afghani indica

 cerebral, alert

 woodsy, fresh

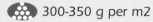 300-350 g per m2

SAGE stands for Sativa Afghani Genetic Equilibrium, but also describes the aroma of this interesting hybrid. SAGE's mother is a native Californian called Big Sur Holy, a sativa with a long finishing time but strong mold and bug resistance. She is combined here with a chunky Afghani indica selected for its extreme characteristics—hardiness, tight internodal structure, and fast finishing time—and grown from seed for cross breeding.

The vigorous growth, elegant leaves, straight growth pattern, and hefty weight of the Afghani balance with the pleasant, mentally alert and thoughtful sativa high, which continues to be satisfying with repeated use. A fulfilling equilibrium of the parental lines, this plant deals well with challenging conditions, and will usually be the last plant standing in a stressed garden. SAGE holds her color and resists mite infestation.

The SAGE flavor is "old-school," reminiscent of the days when Colombian and Thai stick were still primo. The aroma is like the wild sage native to the sativa mama's California homeland. This fresh smell is also a helpful factor for the stealth grower—the odor doesn't readily give away its source. Even without charcoal filters, trained noses may not recognize the scent as weed.

SAGE responds well to topping and is also amenable to the bend technique because the branches hold the rubbery quality of the Afghani papa. This plant likes to grow large, so it works great in beds as a larger plant but is too wily for a sea of green method. Hash made from this variety won first place in the 1999 Cannabis Cup and scientific analysis by an unaffiliated testing facility reported that SAGE's THC content is over 20 percent, ranking in the top 3 varieties tested.

Sensi Star

 I

 56-63 days

 350-450 g per m2

SOG

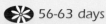 stabilized indica strains with a hint of sativa

 strong body stone possibly cerebral

 pungent

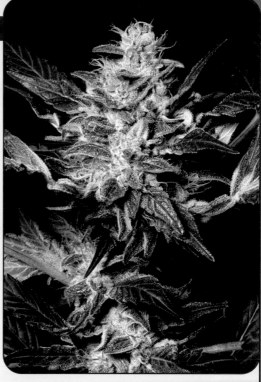

photo credit: Eric K and Paradise Seeds

Sensi Star is a great indoor plant, producing powerful, resinous, and very compact buds. Although mostly indica, she retains a complex high that affects the mind as well as the body. Introduced in 1995 by Paradise, this strain's stability was improved in 1997 to deliver a strong plant with big fan leaves and nice thick buds.

Sensi Star works well in a sea of green set-up with 20 plants per square meter potted close together. It is best to let them vegetate for 2 weeks before entering the 12/12 light cycle. If the strong side branching is allowed to remain and flower, she needs a little extra space. Hydroponic and soil methods are equally suitable. Prospects for gardening this plant outdoors are good in temperate zones, where she will reach approximately 6 feet (2 meters) and produce an average of 400 grams in a successful season.

This headstrong indica produces rock hard colas that have a lemony scent and taste. Some smokers find the buzz to be a very strong body stone, while others report a high with more energetic, cerebral properties as well as a body sensation. THC levels have been reported at 20 percent for this variety, making it a one-hitter quitter. CBD has been measured at .9 percent.

Sensi Star has earned her name, with prizewinning performances in the 1999 *Highlife* Cannabis Cup where she won first place in the bio indoor category. She claimed first prize in the same year at the *High Times* Cannabis Cup for the indica category, returning in 2000 to take 2nd place in the *High Times* Cup's indica category.

Shark Shock

I

40-45 days in early Oct out

500-600 g per m2

White Widow x Skunk #1

stoney

fruity

Shark Shock grows into a densely compacted white skunk with extreme aromas and a high that dazes the smoker with pleasure. Resulting from a cross of the infamous White Widow with the Skunk #1, Shark Shock is a mostly indica plant that develops hairs ranging in color from flaxen to rust and shines with gleaming crystals.

A cross known by many aliases, Shark Shock shares genetic heritage with Peacemaker and Great White Shark. The buds are compact and heavy along very strong and uniform branches. If grown to full size, it can get as a large as 9 feet (3 meters) in height and widens to a traditional evergreen shape. Under controlled indoor growing settings, the average height is 4 feet (1.2 meters).

This plant will produce great finger hash and excels in its fruity taste and intensely stoney effects. Indoors, expect a happily brief flowering cycle of 40-45 days that can yield up to 500-600 grams per square meter. Outside, this plant finishes in the Northern hemisphere in late September or early October; in the Southern hemisphere March to early April is harvest time. While not a temperamental variety, growers should take care not to overfertilize in order to reap the best results.

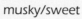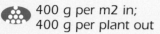

Sheherazade

IS 75/25

56 days

400 g per m2 in;
400 g per plant out

Afghani x mostly sativa SE Asian plant

body relaxation

musky/sweet

SOG

Named for the heroic woman in the Arabian legend, *The Thousand and One Nights*, Paradise's Shererazade will take considerably less time than the title implies, finishing in about 56 nights. In the legend, the character Sheherazade saves her own life using her exceptional storytelling skills that awe the King into sparing her life and eventually taking her as his Queen. The variety bearing her name will spellbound you with the promise of her potent, musky-sweet flowers, possibly making her the queen of your crop.

Sheherazade reveals her Afghani-Kush traits in appearance and other growth indications, but the one-quarter sativa shines through in the quality of the high, which is dynamic and long lasting. The overall sensation is one of bodily relaxation: warm, caressing and deep, but may register on a cerebral level too, encouraging some intriguing yarn spinning of your own. The flavor is as heavy and sweet as the enticing odor.

Perfect for a sea of green set-up, Sheherazade stays on the short side and hardly branches or stretches at all. She likes to be a one-stem plant with a big top flower cluster. In a standard sea of green, Sheherazade will yield an average of 400 grams per square meter. Outside, she can grow to a maximum height of 6 feet (2 meters) with few leaves and many budding locations along her branches. She is recommended for outdoor grows around the 50th parallel N.

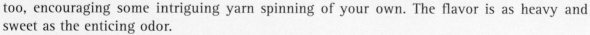
photo credit: Eric K and Paradise Seeds

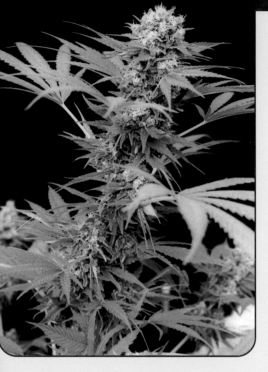

Shit

 I

 45-50 days in late Sep out

 550-650 g per m2

 Skunk & Afghani

mellow

fruity, strong

When it comes to Shit, Mr. Nice growers were having some fun with names. While Mr. Nice breeder Shantibaba admits that it may only be adolescent humor, he still gets a kick from having a variety that people ask for by ordering the Nice Shit. A classic original Skunk/Afghani hybrid, this strain is a profusely branching plant with large sticky buds. It is easy as pie for all to grow whether indoors, greenhouse, or outdoors is the location. First time cultivators will find this one a good starter variety. Water plentifully–this variety likes conditions better wet than dry.

According to Mr. Nice, this variety is "the shit." A Christmas tree of a pot plant, Shit stays medium in height but fills out well. Hairs range from light yellow to red to brown at finish. Even as a multiple branch plant, you will be satisfied with the finishing time of under 7 weeks indoors. Yields can be substantial, ranging between 550-600 grams per square meter. The buzz is mellow and even, giving you sweet skunky breath. The high can last a long while, but in moderation, will not make you so stoned that it disrupts typical everyday activities.

Shiva Skunk

 I

 45-55 days

 up to 450 g per m2

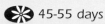 SOG

 Skunk 18.5 (f-3a) x Northern Lights 5

 stoney

 pungent and sweet

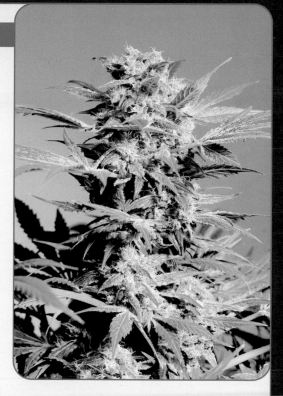

Shiva Skunk shows the excellent vigor of a well-chosen hybrid, making it a snap to grow. Shiva (related to the original Shiva/Shanti) was a selected Afghani type that was part of the Sensi Seed gene bank in the 1980s. When the Seed Bank and Sensi Seeds merged in 1990, the original Shiva mother was replaced by the top Northern Lights strain - NL 5. The Skunk 18.5(f-3a) originates from the Skunk # 1, but is a backcrossed line. A combination of two power plants, Shiva Skunk retains the sweet pungency of her Skunk parent, but has the higher yield and more profuse resin content of the Northern Lights family. While suitable only for an indoor grow in Holland's wet weather, this variety may do well outdoors in the more forgiving weather of Spain or California. Most indoor methods will give pleasing results, including a sea of green–style garden. Sensi's Cannabis Castle growers recommend hydroponic methods for a clean and easy growing experience.

Shiva Skunk is a potent, quick indica that has become popular with commercial growers. Very reliable and stable, this strain is hardly skunk and very Northern Lights in appearance. As with the original NL 5, you can expect that your plants will not stretch very much but stay short with dense, super-resinous indica flowers. You can practically leave your scissors behind when harvesting, the foliage is so minimal. Delivering a sweet, fragrant smoke, Shiva Skunk will yield sweet, spicy buds that give a psychedelically stoney buzz. A kaleidoscope and some Shiva Skunk is a recipe for hours of entertainment.

Cannabis Attractions: The Hash, Marijuana & Hemp Museum

Back in the mid-1980s, two brothers owned the Goa coffeeshop. Together with the married brother's wife, they acquired a building along the canals in central Amsterdam, and came up with the idea of creating a museum devoted to cannabis. After gathering display cases and setting up the building to house a museum, they recruited marijuana columnist and activist Ed Rosenthal to serve as curator.

After three weeks of intensive work filling the cases and walls with cannabis curios and memorabilia from Ed's private collection as well as from many other sources, the museum publicly announced its official opening on Christmas Eve 1984. The gala opening received international press attention but unfortunately the limelight also caught the attention of the Dutch government. The Minister of Justice took particular offense to the museum on the grounds that it incited people to use cannabis.

Although the founders argued that the museum's purpose was educational, the fledgling institution came under legal scrutiny. Rosenthal and the female owner, whose name appeared on the building's paperwork, were forced to defend the museum on the grounds that display does not equal advocacy in the Dutch court system. In the face of opposition, the brothers decided to withdraw from the project. The museum temporarily foundered, but speedily recovered when Ben Dronkers of Sensi Seed Bank stepped in to support the project.

Feeling that the preservation of cannabis culture was an essential contribution worthy of the fight, Dronkers bought the property in which the museum was housed and took over management of the collection, which was renamed the Hash, Marijuana & Hemp Museum. Rosenthal and the female owner were eventually indicted, but eight years after the controversial

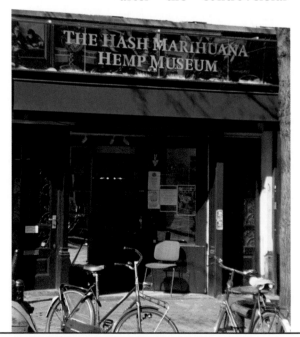

opening, the court cases were settled in favor of the museum.

The female founder and Rosenthal were found guilty and fined for possession of under an ounce of marijuana. They actually possessed much more than that, several pounds—all of which had been sprayed with rubber cement to render it toxic for consumption, and then placed on display after receiving approval from the police.

Today, Dronkers and his sons, Alan and Ravi, work together to maintain an interesting collection of marijuana and hemp history and culture. With the assistance of U.S. activists Chris Conrad and Mikki Norris, the museum's collection was updated and reorganized in 1999 to incorporate modern aspects of cannabis, including an exhibit on the U.S War on Drugs. Since its inception, the Hash, Marijuana & Hemp Museum has sought to be a repository for the rich history of this outlaw plant. While cannabis culture has been driven underground in most parts of the world, Amsterdam provides an environment where this plant's fascinating journey can be recorded. The museum serves an educational purpose, spreading information and dispelling the myths created in an age of cannabis hysteria and censorship.

On average, 65,000 visitors from all over the world stop in at the museum each year.

Given its success, the museum is currently relocating to a larger space just down the street from its current location at Oudezijds Achterburgwal 148. With the move to a new location, a considerable expansion of the collection is underway. The extensive permanent exhibit will be updated to include a display of antique hemp-processing equipment, along with the diverse items it now features, which include books and posters from the U.S. reefer madness period, a grow room with flowering plants, a collection of hemp clothing from minority and tribal peoples of Southeast Asia and Eastern Europe, antique containers that held homeopathic cannabis extracts, and a display of pipes from around the world. Rotating profiles on cannabis personalities, from the famous artist and cannabis afficionado Simon Vinkenoog to present day pioneers, such as Jack Herer will also be added to the attractions.

The Hash, Marijuana & Hemp Museum acquires items for the collection through purchase or donation, and charges a modest admission fee. While going toward the upkeep of the museum, marijuana enthusiasts can also feel satisfied that a portion of the museum's profits are contributed to worthy causes, including support for the harm reduction initiatives of Rotterdam cleric, Reverend Visser, fiber hemp research, hemp events, and legalization efforts.

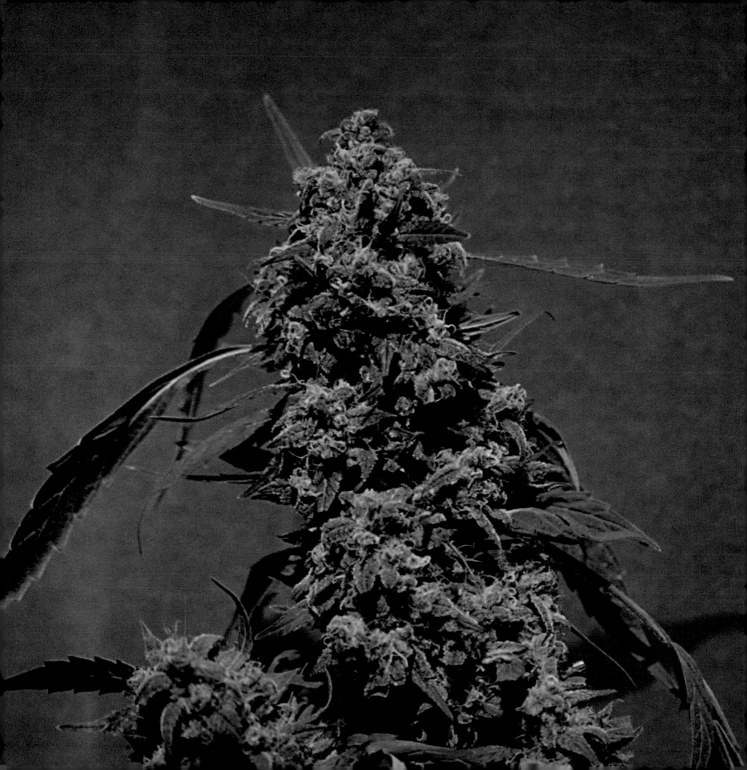

Silver Blue

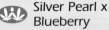

 60/40

 56-63 days

varies

SOG

Silver Pearl x Blueberry

even head-body, psychedelic

citrus, berry

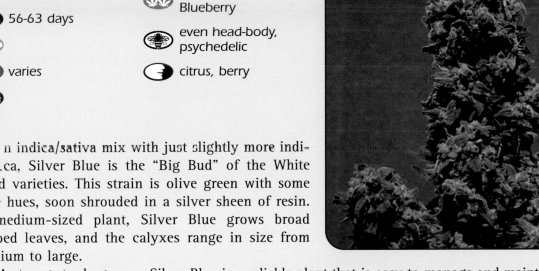

An indica/sativa mix with just slightly more indica, Silver Blue is the "Big Bud" of the White weed varieties. This strain is olive green with some blue hues, soon shrouded in a silver sheen of resin. A medium-sized plant, Silver Blue grows broad shaped leaves, and the calyxes range in size from medium to large.

A strong sturdy grower, Silver Blue is a reliable plant that is easy to manage and maintain in all growing environments. Homegrown Fantaseeds recommends this tough gal for a successful novice experience. After smoking this fine grass, the experienced grower will also be happy to include Silver Blue in his or her garden. An especially good choice for those who favor hydroponics methods, this plant has a high bud-to-stem ratio that makes it a quick manicure at the end of the day.

The mixture of Silver Pearl and Blueberry genetics deliver a plant with a strong aromatic smell and a slightly tart, citrus-berry flavor. A smooth smoke, Silver Blue delivers a full spectrum high, often verging on the hallucinogenic. A great party weed, Silver Blue might put you to sleep if you overindulge.

Silver Haze

 50/50

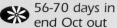 56-70 days in
end Oct out

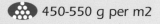

 Skunk, Northern
Lights & Haze

 even head-body

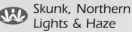 pine, fruit

450-550 g per m2

Silver Haze comprises some of the most commercially recognized strains in the uncivilized world: Skunk, Northern Lights and Haze. It is an excellent breed that shows uniformity in its growth and harvests a top yield with heavy resin production.

A complex hybrid, this variety is in the cutting edge of practical Haze hybrids. Silver Haze shows promising resistance to mold and can be harvested later when everything else has finished. Outdoors, this variety finishes in late October or early November when grown at temperate latitudes. As with most Haze crosses, this variety can grow to be a giant, but can maintain a suitable height for indoor growth if vegetative time is kept to a minimum. Indoor growers should also keep the air circulating around these plants for the best outcome. While not the easiest plant to grow, it is possible for all levels of growers to have success.

The resin glands have very thick heads perched atop a short neck. The airy sativa buds become more compact as they finish, and take on a menthol-pine scent and a mixture of fruit and fresh alpine in the flavor. When burned, this bud can take on a slightly ammonia tone. The buzz is strong but clear, and can be smoked all day without losing its effect.

Silver Pearl

 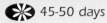

 S I

 45-50 days

Early Pearl, Skunk
 18.5 (f3-a) &
Northern Lights 5

 psychedelic

380 g per m2

sweet

SOG

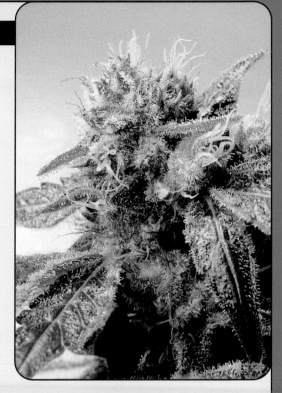

Silver Pearl is the dream child of Northern Lights, a Skunk #1 backcross, and Early Pearl. A true pearl of the pot kingdom, this strain manages to gift wrap all your favorite characteristics of its 3 parents and deliver them in 7 weeks or less.

The Early Pearl parent comes from the U.S. where it was developed in the 1970s and added to Sensi's stable in the early days of the breeding program. A fast-finishing outdoor variety, Early Pearl was a sweet, mostly sativa strain with excellent mold resistance. Northern Lights 5, one of the super Afghani's, has become a building block at Sensi's Cannabis Castle due to it's great uniformity and compact buds. Skunk 18.5 is a Skunk #1 backcross that is consistent and has a high calyx-to-leaf ratio.

Silver Pearl keeps the super fresh, honey flavor of its Early Pearl kin, combined with the consistency, quick finish, and low leaf count of the Northern Lights and Skunk. A short, indica plant type with dense, frosty flowers and few, wide-fingered leaves. Silver Pearl is easy to grow giving excellent indoor results and also performing in the greenhouse. Sea of green or larger plants are suitable, but Sensi prefers the ease and efficiency of the hydro grow. Silver Pearl handles stress with grace, almost never leading to hermaphrodites. The high is energetic and borders on hallucinogenic, a great wake and bake buzz if you want to tingle throughout your day.

Winner, *High Times* Cannabis Cup mixed indica/sativa category 1994

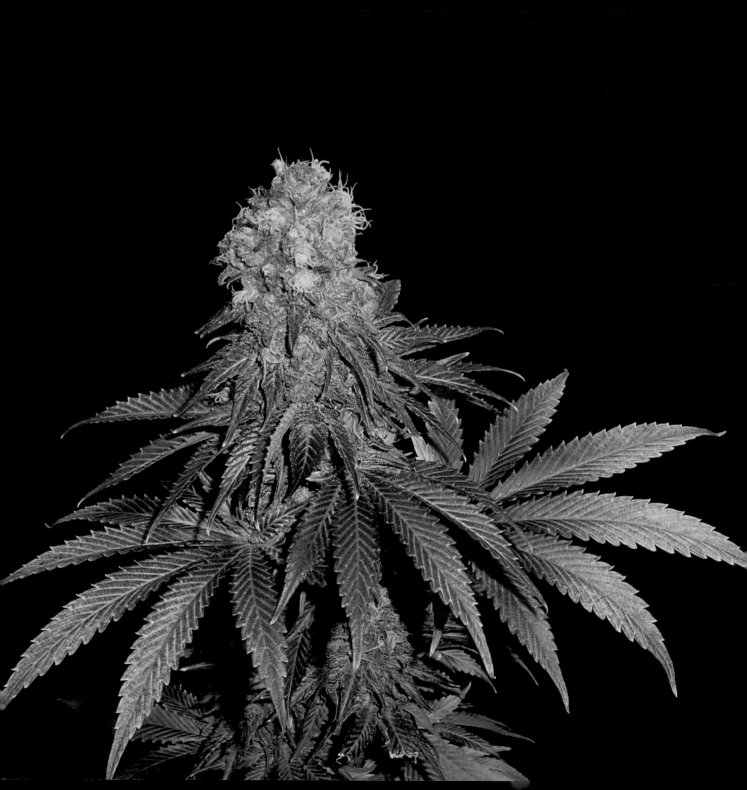

Soma A+

 I

 56 days

 min 12-15 g per plant in 1 gal. pot

 Super Skunk x Big Skunk Korean x Afghani x Afghani Hawaiian

physically relaxing

spicy

SOG

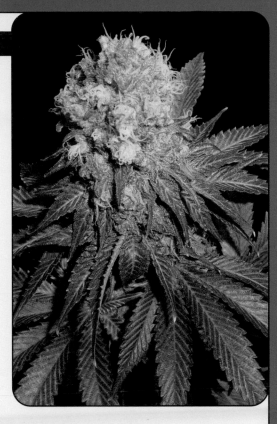

Soma A+ may become the pet of the class. Short to medium in height, this mostly indica strain displays the bushy structure and colas so compact that it has been nicknamed "Rock Bud." She is a good sea of green plant since height and branching are easy to manage. With an extended vegetation period, Soma A+ can be coaxed into a larger plant, and will perform well while still being short enough to stay inconspicuous in an outdoor garden.

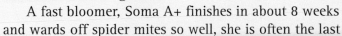

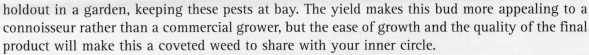

A fast bloomer, Soma A+ finishes in about 8 weeks and wards off spider mites so well, she is often the last holdout in a garden, keeping these pests at bay. The yield makes this bud more appealing to a connoisseur rather than a commercial grower, but the ease of growth and the quality of the final product will make this a coveted weed to share with your inner circle.

At maturity, Soma A+ develops sugary red leaves reminiscent of autumn's best maples. As the mostly indica genetics would lead you to expect, the buzz is relaxing to the body and mind, and good for contemplation or napping on rainy day afternoons. Better as a day ender than a day starter, Soma A+ provides medicinal quality cannabis with healing properties for what ails you, whether physical, psychological, or spiritual in nature.

Paradise Seeds:

Paradise Seeds was founded in 1994 after ten years of experience with growing cannabis and developing quality strains. Back then, our seeds found their way into the hands of people at a local coffeeshop, Lucky Mothers, in Amsterdam. Nowadays, our strains are known the world over and our seeds are distributed in shops and on the internet in many countries. Paradise Seed's aim is in general to create better weed varieties, therefore we maintain strict selection criteria on certain characteristics. Taste, potency and growth patterns are important to us. To satisfy the wishes and needs for growers, smokers and medical patients, it is important to have consistent quality, so this is what we strive for. Our plants are grown on soil organically to give the seeds all ingredients needed for a good start. We now have a large grow space that allows us to test and do research on genetics we consider valuable, allowing us the best tools to do what we love—develop superb weed.

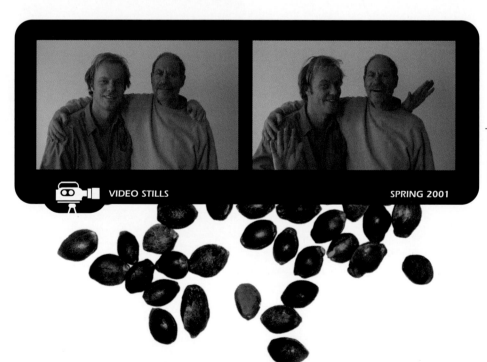

VIDEO STILLS   SPRING 2001

Luc of Paradise Seeds pals around with Ed Rosenthal in Amsterdam

Serious About Seeds

The breeder behind Serious Seeds is Simon. He studied biology at one of the universities in Amsterdam and was always a non-smoker. Then, while traveling though Africa after completing his studies in 1986, he discovered the merits of smoking pure marijuana as opposed to the hashish or marijuana laced tobacco joints commonplace in Europe. From that moment on he started collecting seeds. When he arrived back in Holland, he immediately started growing those seeds out and crossing what he thought were the best plants. Contacts with other growers gave him access to different plants from which he also selected the best ones.

Simon worked for some time at Sensi Seeds and still has a good relationship with the people behind Sensi, Ben and Alan Dronkers. Simon left Sensi, starting his first company in partnership with some American breeders, but then branched out on his own shortly afterward to form Serious Seeds. It has always been a Serious policy to have the products grown from the different seeds available to try out in some of the best coffeeshops in Amsterdam. The "Greenhouse" and the "Dampkring," as well as the "Blue Bird" and "Dread Rock" can be counted on to have some genuine Serious weed on hand for sampling. Serious has always been a small company and prefers to stay like that. With a love for breeding, growing and smoking, Simon works to develop new and interesting plants as well as improving on the classic varieties already offered—not only for business, but for the personal pleasure of quality cannabis.

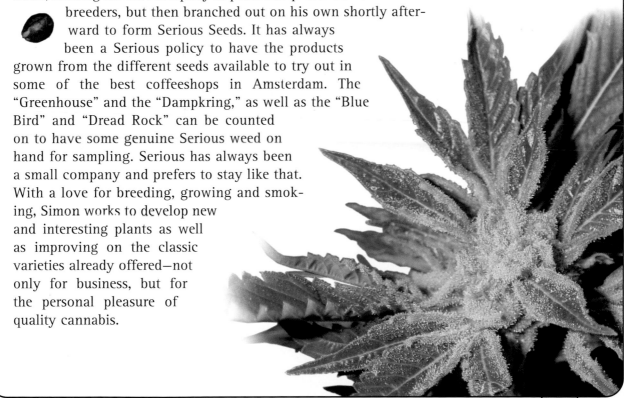

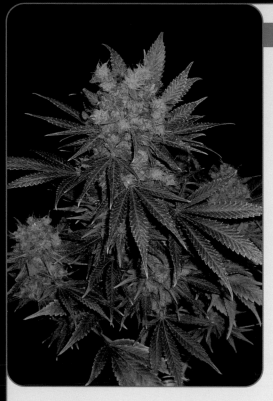

Somango

 63-70 days in

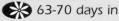

 Jack Herer x Big Skunk Korean

 cerebral, alert

 mango

min 15-20 g per plant in 1 gal. pot

Somango blends the multiple hybrid Jack Herer with Big Skunk Korean to form the fruitiest of all Soma's strains. Previously known by Soma #5, this complex cross was renamed for its tropical mango aroma and flavor.

Somango is optimal as a multiple branch plant, since its genetics encourage long side branches and a height on the taller side. A sea of green method can still be undertaken, but branching and height will need to be controlled. Soma prefers to grow on soil indoors with fully organic nutrients, but other media will also give satisfactory results. As it matures, the leaves shade to purple and the buds become covered in a carpet of crystals that makes fine finger hash. While a moderate yielder, Somango's bud possesses sublime qualities.

The fragrant and tasty Somango smoke delivers a buzz that is very uplifting and mentally stimulating in its effects. You can smoke this pot without turning into a remote control-wielding couch potato. Euphoric and alert, Somango is a good choice for shifting mental attitude and is a good companion to all of your favorite creative undertakings.

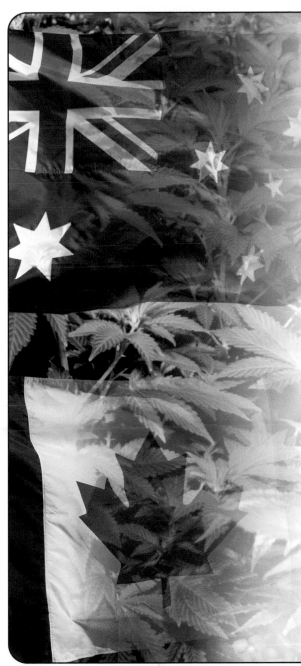

KOG

"I'm just a little bloke having a go against the whole system. Australian farming has never been easy. Right from the start, farmers of any kind have had to struggle to make a meager living off the land. For the last 20 years, there has been one crop that many farmers have dared to grow—a crop that has helped out thousands of struggling farmers. That plant is marijuana. I've been growing the Old Mother Sativa outdoors for 18 years now, and I also run Greengrass Publishing. A few years ago, I wrote the outlaw classic, *Marijuana A Grower's Lot*. Even though it is a crime to grow marijuana in most places around the globe, there are no victims. The law books classify it as a crime against society. To that I say, 'Up the revolution!'"

Doc Bush

Doc Bush Seeds is a speck of a company. Based upon the single belief that ganja should be everywhere, Doc Bush feels that seeds are the perfect means to overgrow the governmentals. "Doc" earned his nickname the old-fashioned way—two green thumbs and a dedication to the goddess of cannabis. Over the past few years, Doc has served near the front lines, spreading cannabis in every direction. More recently, the duty has included serving the compassion clubs and Section 56 stakeholders in Canada. Doc Bush Seeds does not produce a wide range of cross-breeds or hybrids. As Doc says, "I like to do one thing very well . . . the rest is up to you."

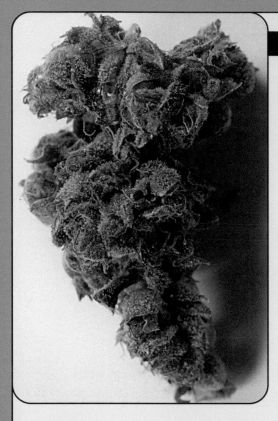

Special Haze

 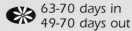

 63-70 days in
49-70 days out

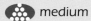

 Nevil's Haze x
KC 606

 cerebral, clear

floral

medium

While most of KC's varieties are designed to grow out in nature, this variety was intended for indoor cultivation. The child of a cross between Nevil's Haze and KC 606, Special Haze retains many of the growth characteristics and effects that have given the Haze so much name recognition.

Special Haze is a giant girl, outpacing most plants in height. The internode spacing is beneficially closer than many other Haze crosses, giving more budding sites. An early flowering plant, Special Haze requires minimal if any vegetative time, and is often placed directly into a 12/12 lighting cycle as soon as it has rooted. Not well-adapted to a sea of green style garden, this strain does best with plenty of space and good soil, grown with its branching intact.

The cross with KC 606 has given this variety a shorter flowering time, but indoors it will still require 9-10 weeks. This plant should only be attempted in an outside garden by those who live in the tropics, where flowering requires $2\frac{1}{2}$ months to produce mature flowers. If you've had the chance to taste the distinct wildflower nuance of the Haze varieties, you will know why this variety is called special. The Haze flavor is intact, as is the high, which is thoughtful and relaxing without being sedating.

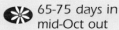

 S I

 65-75 days in mid-Oct out

 Slyder x Western Winds

 cerebral

spicy, sandalwood

325-425 g per m2

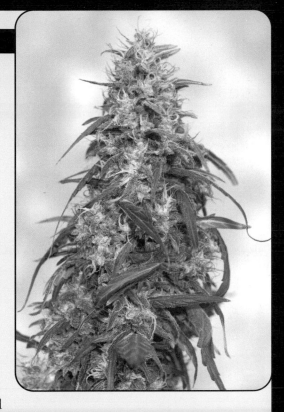

Special K is a sativa/indica hybrid of a Haze-influenced pure sativa named Western Winds and an Afghani/Northern Lights indica named Slyder. Western Winds and Kali Mist share genetic heritage, while Sagarmatha's Slyder is sibling to Serious Seeds' Chronic. Taken together, this Haze sativa and Afghani indica merge into a plant that is tall, with large girth and giant calyxes.

While she may seem a little lanky at first, Special K fills out her height and wide-reaching branches with elongated buds for a pleasing yield. Buds are long and skinny thanks to the presence of indica. She was specifically developed for indoor gardens, but can be grown successfully in the milder regions of the U.S.

Special K produces a quick stone that is cerebral with a psychedelic edge. This high often begins with an indica buzz that goes straight to the eyelids. Once the initial sensation equalizes, you may find yourself googly with the trippy, up vibe Special K invites. This high is long lasting and adventureful. Move over Wheaties—wake and bake with a bowl of Special K for the new millennium Breakfast of Champions.

Mardi Grass Festival, Nimbin, Australia

When Injustice
Becomes Law,
Resistance can be
FUN!
END PROHIBITION
NGA
Get
real
LET IT GROW

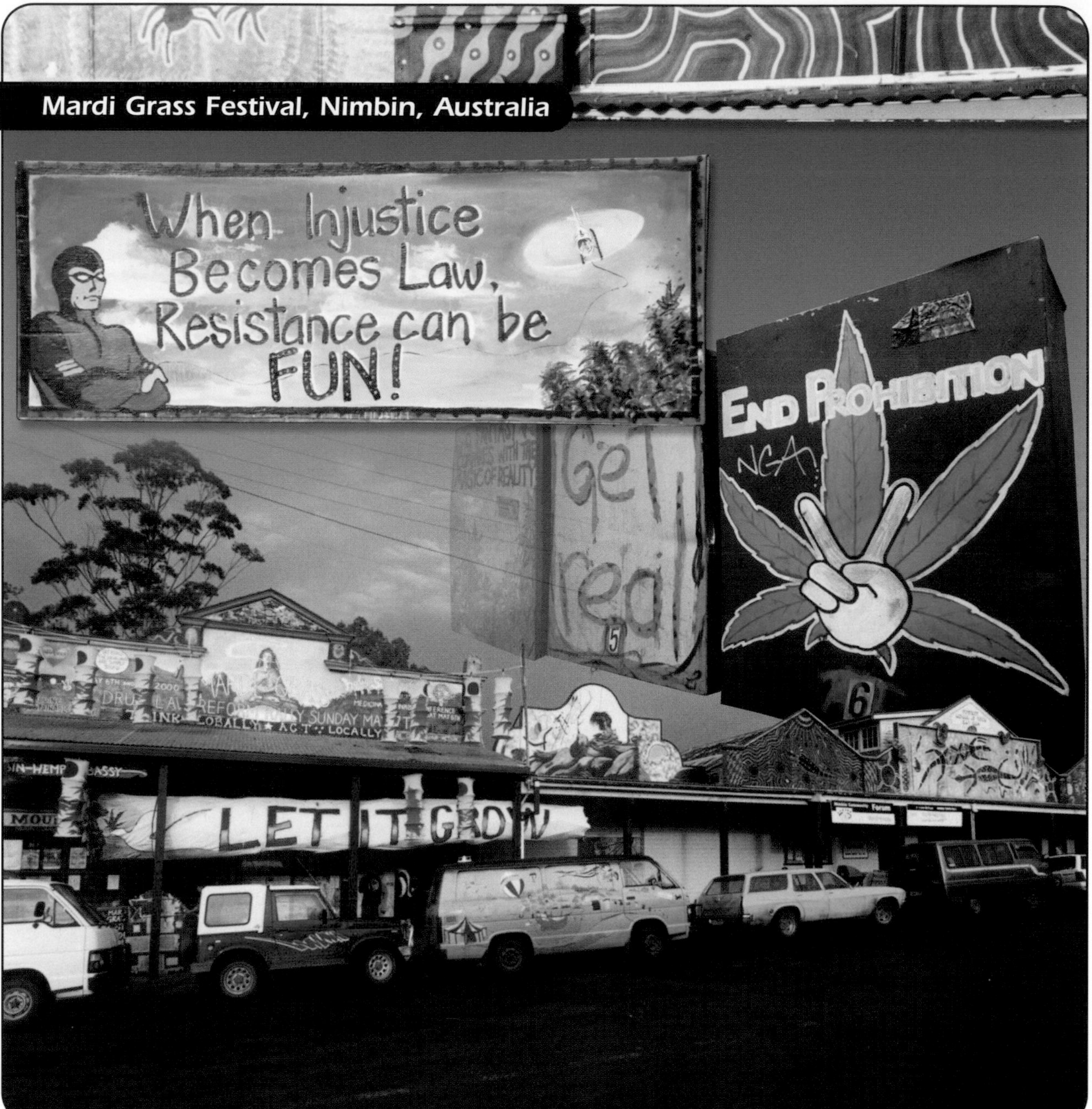

photo credit: Barge

Spice

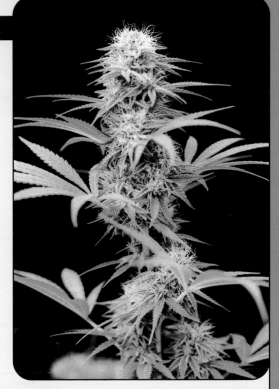

 SI

 49-63 days in
mid-Oct out

 Hawaiian indica x
Hawaiian sativa

 sleepy

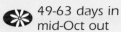 spicy

480-600 g per m2

SOG

Spice's pedigree has blossomed out of an indica/sativa union from the islands of Hawaii. This Aloha State resident was brought to Hawaii from a Kona traveler who collected seed in Asia. He passed the genetics on to Shantibaba, Mr. Nice breeder, back in 1984, since which time it has been selectively bred and further stabilized.

Spice grows with perfectly straight posture to a stately height of 6-9 feet (2-3 meters) outdoors. The large fan leaves acquire a purple aura as the plant finishes, and the thick stem makes staking less critical. The fiery red hairs that form on the colas upon finish give you a hint that she is a sassy smoke. Spice's colas are tight with a banana-shaped curve. Good indoors, this pole pot will fit neatly in a sea of green set-up. This strain is a rapid grower with light branching and an open structure that allows for maximum air flow, making it possible to grow larger plants as well.

You will not be disappointed with the higher than average 480-600 grams per square meter that Spice is capable of delivering. The cured bud has a kick of flavor that is flush with exotic fruit tastes. The smell of the smoke is also quite aromatic and incense-like. This smoke can be dizzying, with an electric edge that may lock you into its powerful physical buzz. Indulging heavily may leave you dozing before you know it.

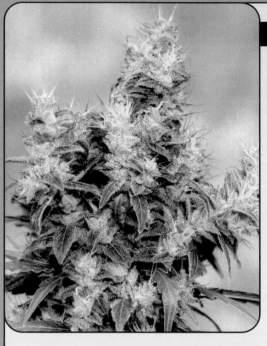

Stonehedge

 I S

 65 days in
mid-Oct out

 350 g per m2
20-30 g per bud

SOG

 Cambodian
California &
Western Winds

 mellow, body high

spicy and sweet

Stonehedge was named to suggest one of the seven wonders of the world, the powerful English symbol that has mystified generations. The name also has a more literal meaning: tended correctly, this tall thick plant would make one hell of a stoney hedge. This variety blends a little Western Winds with a Cambodian California plant that Sagarmatha received from friends in Indiana to create a strong-flavored powerful plant with many beneficial qualities.

Stonehedge does not get extremely leafy, which simplifies manicuring. The colas are very crystally and hard with a terrific bouquet. This plant needs staking in any indoor environment, but performs optimally in a sea of green garden. The aroma and flavor have an acrid, spicy edge to an otherwise floral bouquet. The taste is slightly hashy, with a measure of sweet undertones.

Stonehedge averages in at a short height—only 3 feet (1 meter) indoors. Outdoors, this plant can get quite tall, looking as straight, tall and uniform as a crop of corn. When smoked, Stonehedge creeps into a full buzz, first delivering a little eyedroop, followed by a comfortably relaxed feeling. The slow onset is followed by a slow finish, making for a long-lasting high.

S I

 56-63 days in late Oct out

 Skunk, Northern Lights & Haze

 even head-body

pungent

medium

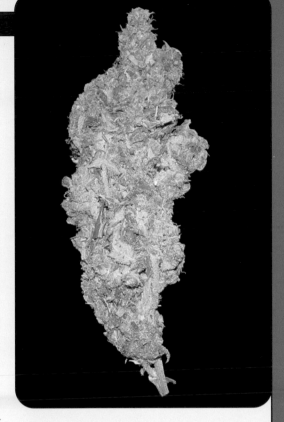

Originally bred by an obscure figure in the Holland marijuana scene, Super Silver Haze has risen to become the Tiger Woods of the pot world. First place winner of three consecutive *High Times* Cannabis Cups for the hydro category (1997, 1998, 1999), Super Silver Haze also claimed first prize in the *High Times* Grand Cup in 1998.

Super Silver combines the stellar genetics of three super plants—the Skunk, Northern Lights and Haze varieties—to deliver an all-around good indoor grower. This variety can also be grown outside in the equatorial zone, approximately between 35 degrees latitude North and South. While she is best grown hydroponically, Super Silver Haze has not let her stardom go to her head. She will produce highly resinous and strongly pungent flowers in most indoor growing set-ups. The colas get pointed on top when mature, and are more open than compact, which makes them harder to manicure but well worth the effort. Sea of green is only recommended for those growers who are masterful at controlling height, since the Haze influence gives this strain a tendency to shoot up.

This variety has a complex nose: a combination of the floral Haze with the sweetness of the Skunk and deep Afghani undertones from the Northern Lights. The flavor is pungent and spicy. Super Silver Haze has a buzz that covers the complete spectrum of effects, with a full-body stone and esoteric, philosophical attributes, making this highly rewarded pot a stash for all seasons.

1st place, *High Times* Hydro Cup 1997, 1998, 1999
1st place, *High Times* Grand Cup 1998

The Dutch Coffeeshop Scene ■ Skip Stone

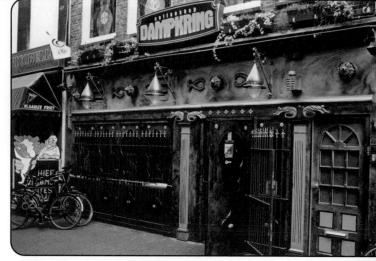

photo credit: Wes Nations

The Dutch have an attitude of tolerance dating back to the 16th century when they forced out the Spanish and their inquisition. Since then, the Dutch make a point of not criminalizing or feigning moral outrage at victimless "crimes." Prostitution, pornography, homosexuality, euthanasia, and soft drug use are all tolerated and integrated into Dutch society. This permissiveness has resulted in Holland becoming a mecca for those who wish to experience the freedom of cannabis culture, and the flowering of a highly successful coffeeshop scene where marijuana and hashish are legally available for purchase by the public.

The "coffeeshop" is a unique Dutch institution. For over 20 years, coffeeshops have operated with quasi-legal status in the Netherlands. Although there is no law that allows for the production and distribution of large quantities of marijuana and hashish, the Dutch tolerate the presence of coffeeshops because they separate the soft drug users from the hard drug dealers. This makes it less likely that someone desiring cannabis would end up purchasing a more dangerous drug, and keeps a whole market away from the illegal drug trade. The Dutch view is that soft drug use is far less damaging to society than imprisoning those who use them.

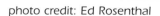

photo credit: Ed Rosenthal

Instead, coffeeshops are regulated by the government on a local level, which requires them to obtain a license and pay taxes. Currently, conferences are being held to decide if a regulatory system can be extended to the growing of cannabis for supplying the coffeeshops. While supply is an obvious necessity for the shops, the cultivation and supply of cannabis remains in a legal shadow, and is still being sporadically prosecuted. Despite the hazy status of growing, the acceptance of cannabis consumption has allowed coffeeshops to flourish with broad acceptance in Dutch society. Marijuana tourists and locals can hang out and toke up in pleasant surroundings with little concern for experiencing the most dangerous side effect of marijuana in most parts of the world: arrest or other legal hassles.

There are approximately 300 coffeeshops operating in Amsterdam, with about 900 total in the entire country of Holland. Coffeeshops may be located almost anywhere including residential areas, but outside of Amsterdam they can be more difficult to find. Some towns have decided NOT to have any coffeeshops and it is their right since they issue the license.

In any coffeeshop you can roll a joint, smoke a pipe or get blitzed from a bong. Most coffeeshops provide complimentary papers and filters or will loan a pipe if you have none. Anyone can sit and smoke in a coffeeshop without buying cannabis there, but as with most establishments, it is necessary to make a purchase, such as a drink or a snack like a tosti (grilled sandwich). Many shops will provide outside seating, and in agreeable weather, it can be an incredibly liberating experience to grab a table and get high outside, much to the amazement of straight tourists! Passing a bong on a crowded sidewalk has the definite flavor of freedom!

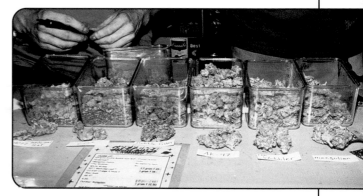

Inside the Grey Area coffeeshop
photo credit: Ed Rosenthal

Since there are so many coffeeshops in Amsterdam, shopping for one that agrees with your taste can be half the fun. Nearly all coffeeshops echo some theme, be it a 60s rock

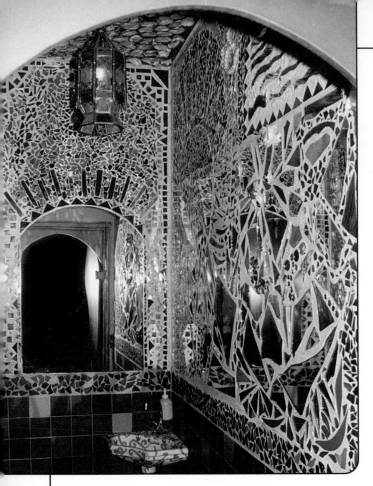

This tile mosaic graces the interior of a Greenhouse coffeeshop. photo credit: Ed Rosenthal

opinion. Some coffeeshops serve coffee and pastries, while others may offer a full menu, prepare specialty items such as smoothies or organic treats, or serve alcoholic beverages. And of course the variety, quality and price of the marijuana and hashish will be key. Location may also be a deciding factor, if a coffeeshop is located close to your home base, or in a neighborhood you particularly enjoy. Most people tend to find a coffeeshop that suits their style, and frequent it regularly.

Tourists are attracted to the larger coffeeshops that advertise, but the locals tend hang out in their neighborhood coffeeshops where the prices are lower. Most Dutch people just pop in to buy some grass then go smoke elsewhere. Coffeeshops usually have a separate counter where they sell cannabis. To buy cannabis in a coffeeshop, just ask for their "menu". It will list both hash and grass with prices. Prices vary according to quantity and quality. Marijuana ranges between 10–20 guilders per gram, and can be purchased by the gram or in 25-guilder (about $12) packages.

Hashish is another story. The most reliable high quality will come from Morocco with several different grades to choose from. Black hash from Afghanistan, Nepal, India or

group or an exotic location. Shops vary greatly in the type of music they play, and the ambiance and amenities they offer, which range from a quite cozy environment of only a few tables to elaborate spaces on multiple floors which may offer couches, television, pool tables or internet access. The available food and beverages may also sway your

Pakistan is available everywhere. But for a real treat check out the Nederhash. It's Dutch hashish made from their hydro or bio plants. As a rule of thumb; the lighter color the Nederhash, the better. The current law limits the amount a person can buy to 5 grams of hash or grass, which is enough for anyone! Many coffeeshops also offer 'space cake' or some other pastry or chocolate dessert laced with marijuana or hashish. Beware! It's better to get space cake "to go," otherwise you might not go anywhere for a very long time!

The Dutch coffeeshop scene is not typical of Europe, although things are beginning to change in the European Union. Belgium and Portugal have now decriminalized cannabis and Germany may be next. Despite the "open" borders, laws and attitudes vary drastically from country to country. The Dutch have clearly demonstrated not only how good marijuana can be, but how it can become an integral part of an enlight-

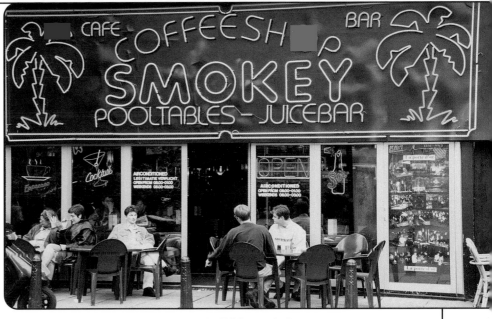

photo credit: Ed Rosenthal

ened society. The Dutch coffeeshop scene is an excellent model for other countries to emulate someday, and for those seeking true freedom, to enjoy now.

Skip Stone is the creator of the *Hip Guide to Amsterdam*, an online resource which includes a guide to Amsterdam's coffeeshops. He has also created a number of other websites including HipPlanet.com, Hippy.com, HipTravel Guide.com and HipForums.com. Skip is the author of *Hippies: From A to Z*, and currently lives in Amsterdam, his favorite hangout.

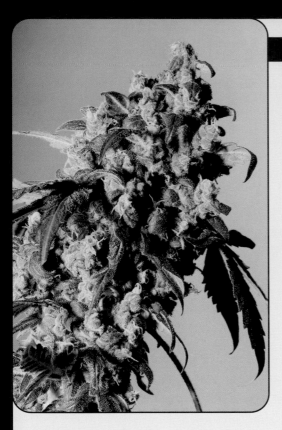

Super Skunk

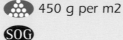

45-50 days in mid-Oct greenhouse

450 g per m2

SOG

Afghani T x Skunk 18.5 (f3a)

even head-body

super skunky smell

Skunkorama! Especially developed for Skunk lovers, this variety reeks with dank skunk odor. Sensi has crossed one of their best skunk lines back to Afghani ancestors, the Afghani T, to create the Super Skunk: a variety with body and beautiful flower formation that is quick and easy to grow.

Successful indoors or for greenhouse gardening in most temperate zones, Super Skunk also fares well in the outdoors, given a mild, arid climate. It is suitable for most standard indoor gardening methods, including the sea of green style. Cannabis Castle growers recommend employing hydroponics for an efficient garden with quick results. The good yield potential and agreeable nature of this strain make it a good selection for beginners and commercial growers alike.

Super Skunk is short to medium in height with wide indica-style leaves and compact flowers. Merely brushing against this plant releases a powerful skunk aroma that fills the grow room, which may require some tact or at least some privacy if guerilla growing. The flavor is dense and sweet, and the buzz flows through the mind and body, although it can lead to lethargy if smoked in quantity.

Winner, *High Times* Harvest Festival 1990

Swazi Safari

 S

 63-84 days in
Oct out

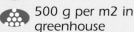 500 g per m2 in
greenhouse

 Skunk #1 (m) x
Swaziland sativa (f)

 cerebral, clear

piney

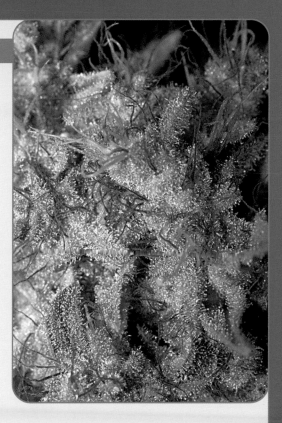

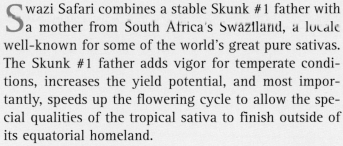

Swazi Safari combines a stable Skunk #1 father with a mother from South Africa's Swaziland, a locale well-known for some of the world's great pure sativas. The Skunk #1 father adds vigor for temperate conditions, increases the yield potential, and most importantly, speeds up the flowering cycle to allow the special qualities of the tropical sativa to finish outside of its equatorial homeland.

A tall, slim plant with scant, light green foliage, Swazi Safari turns to golden tones as the flowers mature. The growth pattern leans toward its mostly sativa heritage, but the buds are exceptionally dense for a sativa. Flowers form clusters at many sites along the branches, yielding an average of 500 grams per square meter when grown in a greenhouse using soil. In a sea of green method, the branching is easy to control, but the yield potential is better when growing methods that encourage multiple budding sites are used.

Swazi Safari has a relatively long finishing time, taking between 9-12 weeks for harvest, but the wait is worth it. The last few days of ripening can add 15-25 percent to the yield and the resin crystals increase exponentially in the race to the finish. With a fresh scent and sweet pine flavor, Swazi Safari is a delicacy that any ganja gourmand will savor. Perhaps more special yet is the luminous quality of the sativa high, leaving the user feeling euphoric yet clear-headed. A truly cerebral pot, Swazi Safari can make any day a little sunnier.

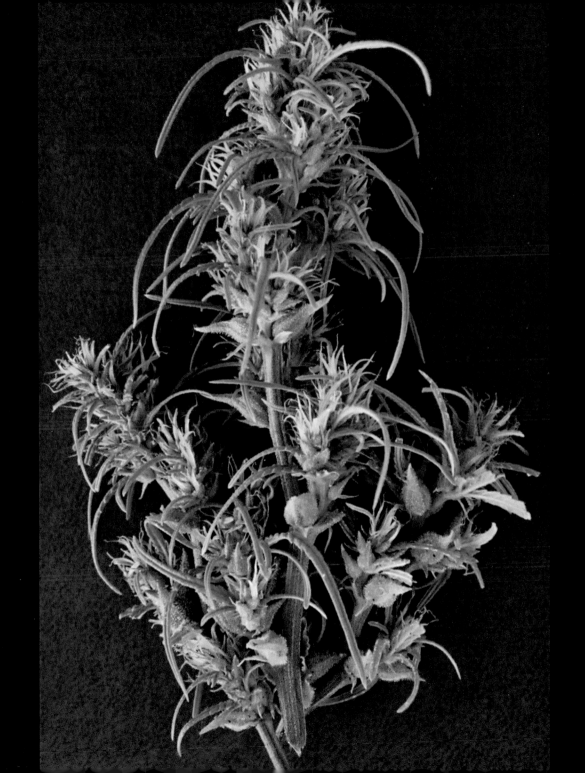

Swazi Skunk

S

 56-77 days in
84-112 days out

 1-2 oz per plant in
20-30 oz per plant
out

 Swazi sativa from the
Pigs Peak Highland

cerebral, alert

earthy, tobacco

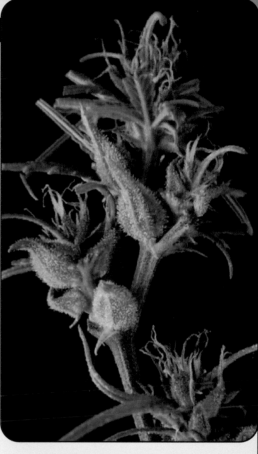

Swazi Skunk is the real thing. Derived from seed stock originally from breeders in Swaziland, this plant has been exclusively inbred—never hybridized— and adapted for indoor use. In South Africa, the potent, seedless bud of this pure sativa began to be called "skunk" locally, which should not be confused with the indica/sativa skunk hybrids of Europe.

This plant has a strong odor like a fine cigar. The smoke is also earthy. It has a taste similar to Durban breeds, with a liquorice aftertaste. The high is energetic and very clear-headed, a good daytime smoke as this pot does not induce heavy or sleepy physical sensations.

Swazi Skunk shows its all-sativa heritage in its appearance, growth patterns, and high. This variety grows to a height between 4-6 feet indoors, and up to 14 feet outdoors depending on conditions and growing time. The branching is extensive with large, slim fan leaves, and compact, sticky buds covered in hair and visible resin glands. Grown outdoors to full size, this plant can yield colas the length of a typical adult's forearm. Indoors, the best plants yield buds up to 8 inches long.

For best results outdoors, Swazi Skunk likes equatorial conditions: warm days (between 70-90 degrees F) and at least 5 months with no frost to grow to its full potential and produce its best yield. It can withstand shorter and cooler summer climates, but will not be able to grow as large and the yield will be diminished as a result. Indoors, a hydroponic system with an ebb and flow minimum is required for success.

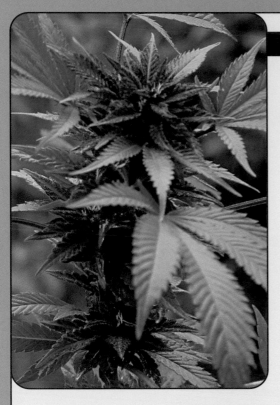

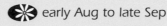
 1S

 early Aug to late Sep

 500 g per plant

 Purple strain x Dutch strain x mystery strain

 clear, physically relaxing

herbal

Sweet Purple is a hybrid of 3 varieties: a purple variety, an early-finishing and large-yielding Dutch variety and a third, mystery strain of strong potency. As the name implies, this strain kept the coloration of the purple parent, while gaining sweetness from the Dutch part of the family. This mostly indica mix was bred by Paradise Seeds in 1999 for outdoor gardens in temperate climates.

Any time a Dutch breeder claims a variety can grow outdoors in Holland, you can bet that she'll stand up to cold, wet climates. Sweet Purple has the additional benefit of resisting mold. These hardy plants grow to a full height of about 8 feet (2.5 meters) and can yield 500 grams per fully matured plant. Sweet Purple shows some variation, and potency can vary from average to "wow" from one plant to another. The coloration also ranges—some plants turn completely purple, while others take on this royal hue on the buds alone.

Sweet Purple has a strong herbal bouquet, and a sweet taste with an iron-like tone to it. The high is a pleasant bodily sensation, but also retains a lucid edge that may increase your sense of concentration.

Ultra Skunk

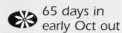

 65 days in
early Oct out

 475 g per m2 with
1000 wpm

SOG

 Big Bud (m) x
Skunk (f)

 cerebral, wandering
mind, creative

sweet, pungent
smell/smooth taste

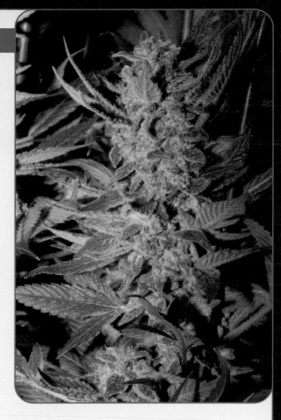

This Big Bud x Skunk cross is a classic hybrid. Although thousands of varieties have been offered since this was created in the 1980s, Ultra Skunk remains one of the most dynamic plants for both indoor and outdoor gardeners. It is strong and vigorous and wants to produce, even under adverse conditions. With champion potency, your focus will quickly pass from the fruity-skunk aroma and seductively smooth draw to your changed attitude toward life—all in just 60 seconds. The high is mind-opening, creative and bordering on the psychedelic.

Ultra Skunk's seeds are f2 generation Skunk x Big Bud, but are the first feminized generation. The plants have a combination of characteristics ranging from the Thai and Mexican parentage of the stabilized Skunk to the Afghani indica parents of Big Bud. This reliably vigorous plant matures in 9-10 weeks indoors and in mid-October (mid season) at mid-U.S. latitude. Ultra Skunk resists early ripening in the South. Your patience in the last weeks of ripening will be well worth it as you witness the glands filling toward the very end of the maturation cycle.

Ultra Skunk is mildly difficult to clone. Once the clones take, this plant is a robust grower, with wide branching and the ability to grow tall. It can be used in a sea of green with pruning to a single stem at forcing and again at 2 weeks. It is excellent for large containers. Outdoor growers can expect a big bush when planted early, and will find it excellent for late planting. Popular among medical users, Ultra Skunk rewards the user with a creative and cerebral high, although the contemplation it encourages may tend to distract from any activites that require focused attention.

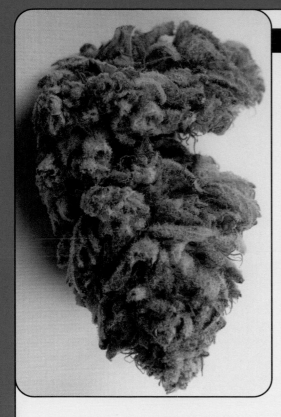

White KC

 I

 42-77 days in 56-70 days out

good

 White Widow, KC special select, KC33, & Afghani-like plant

 body stone, sleepy

fruity

KC has crossed a special select strain of his own with KC 33 and a 1995 White Widow strain, then mixed in an Afghani-like plant to form White KC. This plant has retained the appearance of the White family, growing to a medium height and revealing considerable resin production at maturation.

The cross gave White KC a speedier flowering time, making it suitable for outdoor growing in temperate zones. This variety is not a big fan of the cold, and tends to be particular about frost and other weather conditions. It offers more consistent results when gardening indoors, where it can be grown using any standard method, although trimming those fat, light-blocking leaves is important to maximizing the bud production.

Expect big chunky buds from this indica plant. White KC is also a good choice for the grower interested in processing for hash, given its prodigious output of resin. With a fruity scent, and a soft, subtle fruity flavor, this variety's heavy stone may make you feel like pulling a Rip van Winkle.

KC Brains—Outstanding in His Field

KC has been breeding for almost 20 years. A lover of the outdoor strains, he shoots for the biggest plants he can get. Growing the big girls has been KC's way to show that plant count laws can be used to an advantage. KC likes to grow his personal plants on his roof in big pots. He is currently trying to beat the odds by seeing just how tall he can get his plants to grow. His current goal: "I want to see if maybe 7 meters (about 23 feet) is possible." KC offers a grow tip: "Water your plants with mineral water. They love it. Every plant loves it. It's direct CO_2 to the roots."

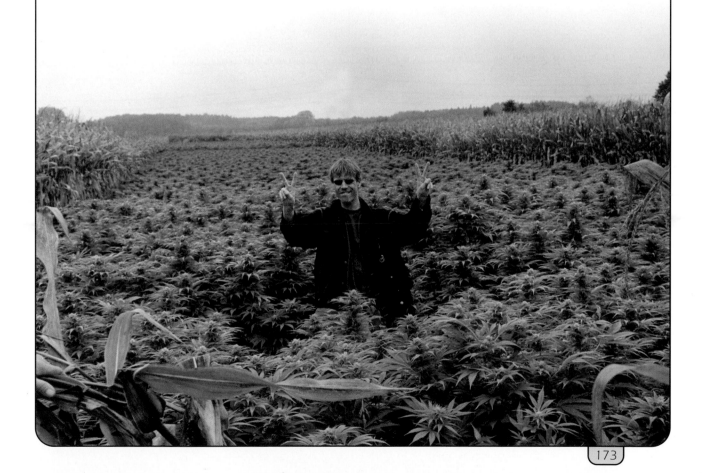

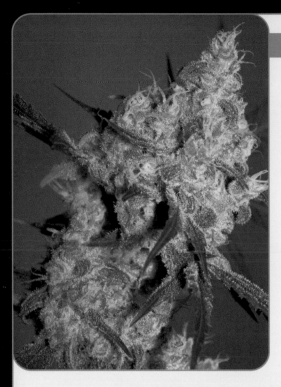

White Russian

 58-62 days

 350-450 g per m2

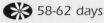 White Widow x AK-47

alert, clear

sweet, pungent

SOG

White Russian combines AK-47 with the White Widow to produce a snowy plant with a pleasantly sweet aroma and a strong, clear high. It was not until much later that Serious Seeds breeder, Simon, became aware of the alcoholic cocktail by the same name.

This easy-to-grow plant works equally well in soil or hydro. Intermediate in size, White Russian is not very leafy, giving it an open canopy that makes it perfect for indoor gardening. This plant is appropriate for a sea of green method. The yield is excellent, with a normal harvest producing 350-450 grams per square meter.

The mottled green colas resemble their indica heritage in size and density, and are typically coated with light tan crystals. At maturity, the hairs turn to auburn. White Russian buds smell sweet and green, with a light undertone of skunk. The sweetness is enhanced in the flavor, although heavier like hash oil rather than lighter like flowers.

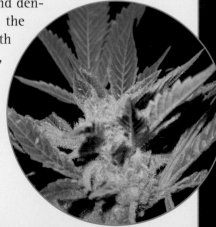

An expansive smoke, White Russian has a clear high with long duration. The effect can be complex, but tends toward wakefulness rather than sleep, and may have some trippy or spacey dimensions: A good afternoon smoke with a cup of coffee when you're ready to kick back and relax.

Overall Winner *High Times* Cannabis Cup 1997
Winner *High Times* Cannabis Cup, Organic Pot 1996

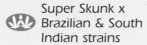

 SI 75/25

 56-70 days

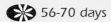

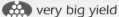 very big yield

SOG

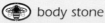 Super Skunk x Brazilian & South Indian strains

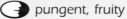 body stone

pungent, fruity

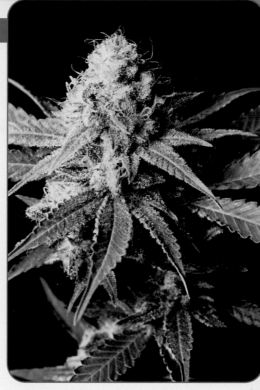

Also known as Peacemaker, the White Shark produces heavy colas with a resin coverage that rivals White Widow. A mostly indica plant, the body buzz is potent, often making this a one-hitter quitter. Also well known for its medical properties, White Shark is a strain of choice for those who suffer from chronic pain.

The Super Skunk, Brazilian and South Indian parents have given White Shark the stereotypical indica appearance, with fat, serrated leaves and dense, chunky colas on a squat, easily manageable plant. The powdery buds develop the traditional Halloween orange hairs that darken to brown as the crop reaches maturity.

While this variety can be grown outside in mild temperate climates where the growing season allows for a 10-week finish, White Shark is recommended as a hydroponic plant indoors. Other methods, including a sea of green–style garden, can also produce winning yields. A serious buzz with a pungent but distinctly fruity taste, this strain is best indulged in when there is time to daze and doze afterwards.

Winner, *High Times* Cannabis Cup 1997

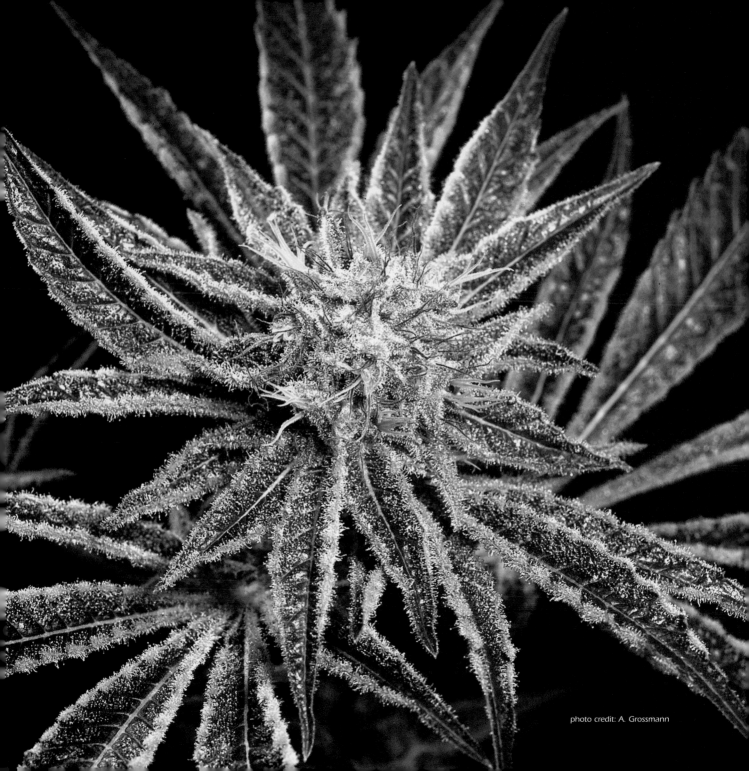

photo credit: A. Grossmann

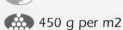

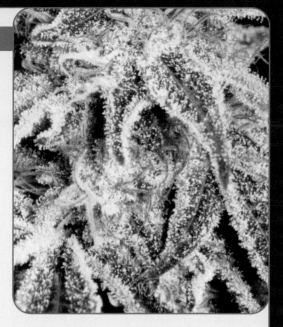

SI 60/40

56-70 days in 70-84 days, or end Oct out

450 g per m2

Indian x Brazilian

even body-head

fresh, fruity, floral

SOG

Since its introduction in 1995, White Widow has become an infamous breed in the world of weed. This variety can be found in almost every coffeeshop in Amsterdam, but while imitation may be the truest form of flattery, the genuine item bears the Greenhouse name.

This variety's reputation has been built on its excellence in smell, flavor, and quality of the high. White Widow has fragrantly fresh pine cone nugs that have a taste bordering between fruit and flowers when smoked. Setting the standard for kind bud, White Widow washes over you with a warm feeling of impending stoniness. While the buzz is strong, it is not sedating, producing a mixture of effects that are both cerebral and physical, but may include both spacy or mildly trippy sensations.

White Widow is a compact plant of medium height. The buds only develop a few amber-colored hairs, but the outrageous crystalline resin production of this plant has become legendary. Inevitably the reputation that precedes it leads some growers to decide that it is over-rated, but many find this variety to be everything they anticipated and more. White Widow has the potential to live up to its reputation when grown adeptly. This strain is recommended for indoor gardening, where water and fertilizer should be administered modestly to avoid mildew and retain the delicious flavors. Greenhouse suggests changing the lighting to 8 hours during the last 2 weeks of flowering in order to halt regrowth on the buds and produce just enough stress to coax out the maximum amount of sticky resin per inch.

1st place, *High Times* Cannabis Cup bio category 1995

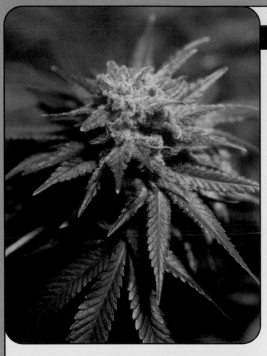

Willy Jack Brainer

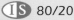 80/20

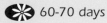 60-70 days

 250 g per plant

 Brain Child backcrossed to Brain Strain

 body stone

pungent scent/ melon taste

SOG

Willy Jack Brainer is a mostly indica cross at only 20 percent sativa. Honed over 15 years of selective breeding, this strain was the result of crossing female pollen from Brain Strain to a cross of Williams Wonder and 1995 Cannabis Cup winner, Jack Herer. The Williams Wonder/Jack Herer hybrid is also known as Brain Child. Brain Child was then backcrossed to Brain Strain, the backbone of the Shadow Seed company. This girl's tomboy name borrows from each part of the three-way cross.

Willy Jack Brainer exhibits desirable growth characteristics, is easy to manicure and is covered in crystals. Willy Jack Brainer was selected for her fruitiness, an unusual flavor for a mostly indica strain. The taste has a deep honeydew coating that covers the back of your throat. The aroma is heavy, one of those telltale smells that makes you put a towel under the door if you don't want the rest of the world to know what you're up to. When done, the odor has hints of a fine premium grade engine oil, that heightens anticipation. She also makes some killer hash oil.

This plant is better suited to an indoor environment and does well in both soil and hydro. Normally reaching about 6 feet (2 meters) in height, it has a generous flower-to-leaf ratio that makes it easy to tame and manicure. The branches are thick and strong enough to support the pleasingly resinous yield. Willy Jack Brainer has the kick-ass buzz you would expect from an indica, complete with couch lock and eyedroop that combine to make napping an appealing post-toke activity.

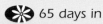
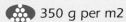

I

 Humboldt California origins

 65 days in

relaxing

woodsy

350 g per m2

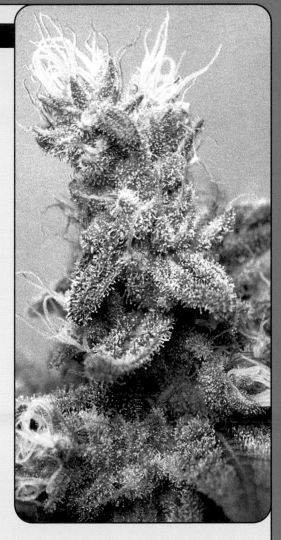

Given to Sagarmatha from a long-time grower in the fabled hills of Humboldt County California, Yumboldt is yummy Humboldt pot. This variety is by and large the epitome of what one expects from pot— it smells exactly like you'd expect pot to smell, and gets you high in that droopy eyelid, sedated, dream-like way that is usually satirized as the stereotypical stoner. Its expansion characteristics make it likely that you'll even get the trademark hacking cough after a big toke.

The taste is like the fine California sinsemilla from the late 1970s. A rich, aromatic and flavorful pot, Yumboldt has a pungent, woodsy smell that carries. If you carry this grass around in your pocket, your friends might start looking expectant and ask when you're going to get around to rolling one up. The buzz is very comfortable and stoney, producing a dreamy demeanor that may phase into actual napping.

A nice chunky indica, Yumboldt produces fat leaves and buds that look and smell like baby pine cones. Flowering can begin after a vegetation period of approximately 2 weeks. This hardy variety is great for the outdoor weather in California, where it used to be known as "Bolt" back in the old days because of the strength and pungency of the buds. Yumboldt also does well indoors, in whatever set-up you prefer, with an average height of 3 feet (1 meter).

Homegrown Fantaseeds ▪ Irish Rose Seed Co. ▪ Jordon of the Islands ▪ KC Brains ▪ Kog's Own S
erious Seeds ▪ Shadow Seed Co. ▪ Soma's Seeds ▪ TH Seeds ▪ African Seeds ▪ Connoisseur Coll
ying Dutchmen ▪ Greenhouse Seed Co. ▪ Greenthumb Seeds ▪ Homegrown Fantaseeds ▪
ank ▪ Nirvana ▪ Paradise Seeds ▪ Sagarmatha ▪ Sensi Seed Bank ▪ Serious Seeds ▪ Shado
oc Bush Seeds ▪ Dr. Atomic ▪ Enterprise Seeds ▪ Federation Seed Co. ▪ Flying Dut
ordon of the Islands ▪ KC Brains ▪ Kog's Own Seeds ▪ Medifarm ▪ Mr. Nice Seed Ban
eeds ▪ TH Seeds ▪ African Seeds ▪ Connoisseur Collection Seed Co. ▪ DJ Short ▪
ed Co. ▪ Greenthumb Seeds ▪ Homegrown Fantaseeds ▪ Irish Rose Seed Co.
aradise Seeds ▪ Sagarmatha ▪ S ensi Seed Bank ▪ Serious Seeds ▪ Shadow See
eds ▪ Dr. Atomic ▪ Enterprise Seeds ▪ Federation Seed Co. ▪ Flying Dutch
ordon of the Islands ▪ KC Brains ▪ Kog's Own Seeds ▪ Medifarm ▪ Mr. Nice
o. ▪ Soma's Seeds ▪ TH Seeds ▪ African Seeds ▪ Connoisseur Collec
utchmen ▪ Greenhouse Seed Co. ▪ Greenthumb Seeds ▪ Hom egrow
r. Nice Seed Bank ▪ Nirvana ▪ Par adise Seeds ▪ Sagarmat ha ▪
onnoisseur Collection Seed Co. ▪ DJ Short ▪ Doc Bush Seed
reenthumb Seeds ▪ Homegrown Fantaseeds ▪ Irish Rose
irvana ▪ Paradise Seeds ▪ Sagarma tha ▪ Sensi Seed Bank
eed Co. ▪ DJ Short ▪ Doc Bush Seeds ▪ Dr. Atomic ▪ Enter
omegrown Fantaseeds ▪ Irish Rose Seed Co. ▪ Jo rdon
Sagarmatha ▪ Sensi Seed Bank ▪ Serious Seeds ▪ Sha dow S
eeds ▪ Dr. Atomic ▪ Enterprise Seeds ▪ Fe deration Seed C
ed Co. ▪ Jordon of the Islands ▪ KC Brains ▪ Kog's O wn Seed
eeds ▪ Shadow Seed Co. ▪ Soma's Seeds ▪ TH See ds ▪ Afri
Federati on Seed Co. ▪ Flying Dutch men ▪ Gr
lands ▪ KC Brains ▪ K og's Own Seeds ▪ M
Shadow Se ed Co. ▪ S o ma's Seeds ▪
Enterprise Seeds ▪ F ederat ic
Irish Rose Se ed C o. ▪ Jo rc
e Seeds ▪ Sag ar
eeds ▪ Connoiss eur
o. ▪ Flying Dutchmen ▪ Gr
lands ▪ KC Brains ▪ Kog's Own S
erious Seeds ▪ Shadow Seed Co. ▪ Som
r. Atomic ▪ Enterprise Seeds ▪ Federation S
ish Rose Seed Co. ▪ Jordon of the Islands ▪ KC Brains ▪ Kc
ank ▪ Serious Seeds ▪ Shadow Seed Co. ▪ Soma's Seeds ▪ TH
nterprise Seeds ▪ Federation Seed Co. ▪ Flying Dutch
ordon of the Islands ▪ KC Brains ▪ Kog's Own Seeds
eeds ▪ Shadow Seed Co. ▪ Soma's Seeds ▪ TH Seeds ▪ African Seeds
ederation Seed Co. ▪ Flying Dutchmen ▪ Greenhouse Seed Co. ▪ Greenthumb Seeds ▪ Hor
edifarm ▪ Mr. Nice Seed Bank ▪ Nirvana ▪ Paradise Seeds ▪ Sagarmatha ▪ Sensi Seed Bank ▪ Ser
o. ▪ DJ Short ▪ Doc Bush Seeds ▪ Dr. Atomic ▪ Enterprise Seeds ▪ Federation Seed Co. ▪ Flying
ordon of the Islands ▪ KC Brains ▪ Kog's Own Seeds ▪ Medifarm ▪ Mr. Nice Seed Bank ▪ Nirva

Company Acknowledgments

We would like to thank the following companies for their contribution to *The Big Book of Buds:*

African Seeds
www.africanseeds.com
seeds@africanseeds.com

Connoisseur Collection Seed Co.
available through:
Seed Bank of Canada
Box 174
2416 Main St.
Vancouver, BC
V5T 3E2 Canada
(604) 251-6316

DJ Short
available through:
The Amsterdam Seed Company of Canada
Box 4253, 349 West Georgia St.
Vancouver, BC
V6B 3Z7 Canada
(604) 728-5617
www.theamsterdam.com

Doc Bush Seeds
136 Sears St. Unit #4
Toronto, Ontario
M4L 1B3 Canada
www.docbushseeds.com
docbush@netscape.com

Dr. Atomic
available through:
Kind Seed Company
Box 233 - 2906 West Broadway
Vancouver, BC
V6K 2G8 Canada
(604) 408-1198
www.kindseed.com
info@kindseed.com

Enterprise Seeds
702 Columbia St.
New Westminster, BC
V4C 6P5 Canada
www.medicalseeds.com

Federation Seed Co.
available through:
The Amsterdam Seed Company of Canada
Box 4253, 349 West Georgia St.
Vancouver, BC
V6B 3Z7 Canada
(604) 728-5617
www.theamsterdam.com

Flying Dutchmen
OZ Achterburgwal 131, PO Box 10952
Amsterdam 1000 EZ
The Netherlands
www.flyingdutchmen.com

Greenhouse Seed Co.
PO Box 75162
Amsterdam 1070 AD
The Netherlands
www.greenhouse.org

Greenthumb Seeds, Canada
Box 37085
Ottawa, Ontario
K1V 0W9 Canada
www.drgreenthumb.com

Homegrown Fantaseeds
mail:
PO Box 3204
Amsterdam 1001 AA
The Netherlands
store:
Fantaseeds Garden
Nieuwe Nieuwstraat 25
Amsterdam 1012 NG
The Netherlands
www.homegrown-fantaseeds.com

Irish Rose Seed Co.
available through:
Marc Emery Seeds
mail:
M.E.
22 East Cordova St. #209
Vancouver, BC
V6A 4GB Canada
(604)-681-4690, fax (604)-681-4687
www.emeryseeds.com

Jordon of the Islands
available through:
Marc Emery Seeds
mail:
M.E.
22 East Cordova St. #209
Vancouver, BC
V6A 4GB Canada
(604)-681-4690
fax (604)-681-4687
www.emeryseeds.com

KC Brains
+31 (65) 473-0608
Fax: +31 (18) 363 6510
www.kcbrains.com

Kog's Own Seeds
P.O. Box 140
Kyogle
NSW 2474
Australia
www.greengrasspub.com.au

Medifarm
available through:
The Amsterdam Seed Company of Canada
Box 4253, 349 West Georgia St.
Vancouver, BC
V6B 3Z7 Canada
(604) 728-5617
www.theamsterdam.com

Mr. Nice Seed Bank
PO BOX 75014
Amsterdam 1070 AA
The Netherlands
www.mrnice.net

Nirvana
Po Box 2108
Zaandam 1500 GC
The Netherlands
+31 (20) 364-0233
www.nirvana.nl

Paradise Seeds
Postbox 377
Amsterdam 1000 AJ
The Netherlands
Tel / Fax +31 (20) 679-5422
www.paradise-seeds.com
info@paradise-seeds.com

Sagarmatha
mail:
PO Box 3717
Amsterdam 1001 AM
The Netherlands
shop:
Marnixstraat 255
Amsterdam 1015 WH
The Netherlands
www.highestseeds.com
info@highestseeds.com

Sensi Seed Bank
PO Box 1771
Rotterdam 3000 BT
The Netherlands
+31 (10) 476-3044
fax: +31 (10) 477-8893
www.sensiseeds.com

Serious Seeds
Postbus 2796
Amsterdam 1000 CT
The Netherlands
www.seriousseeds.com
serious@xs4all.nl

Shadow Seed Co.
available through:
Seed Bank of Canada
Box 174
2416 Main St.
Vancouver, BC
V5T 3E2 Canada
(604) 251-6316

Soma's Seeds
www.somaseeds.nl

TH Seeds
Nieuwendijk 13
Amsterdam 1012 LZ
The Netherlands
www.thseeds.com
hemp@xs4all.nl

African Seeds
Malawi Gold
Swazi Skunk

Connoisseur Collection Seed Co.
Blue Skunk Special

DJ Short
Blueberry
Blue Moonshine
Blue Velvet
Flo

Doc Bush Seeds
Hashmaster

Dr. Atomic
Atomic Northern Lights
Blueberry x Northern Lights
Northern Lights x Bubble Gum

Enterprise Seeds
Americano
Betazoid

Federation Seed Co.
Hawaiian Sativa
Island Sweet Skunk
Mikado
Romulan

Flying Dutchmen
Dutchmen's Royal Orange
Pot of Gold
"The Pure" Skunk #1
The Real McCoy
Swazi Safari

Greenhouse Seed Co.
El Niño
Hawaiian Haze
Nevil's Haze
Super Silver Haze
White Shark
White Widow

Greenthumb Seeds
Huron
Millennium
Niagara
Niagara x Shiva

Homegrown Fantaseeds
Caramella
Eclipse
Haze 19 x Skunk #1
Original Misty
Silver Blue

Irish Rose Seed Co.
Blueberry x Nice

Jordon of the Islands
BC Big Bud

KC Brains
Bahia Black Head
KC 33
Léda Uno
Mango
Special Haze
White KC

Kog's Own Seeds
  Old Mother Sativa
Medifarm
  Max 49
  Ultra Skunk
Mr. Nice Seed Bank
  Black Widow
  Critical Mass
  Devil
  Early Queen
  La Niña
  Medicine Man
  Shark Shock
  Shit
  Silver Haze
  Spice
Nirvana
  Ice
  Master Kush
  Misty
  New Purple Power
Paradise Seeds
  Amsterdam Flame
  Belladonna
  Durga Mata
  Dutch Dragon
  Nebula
  Sensi Star
  Sheherazade
  Sweet Purple
Sagarmatha
  Bubbleberry
  Mangolian Indica
  Matanuska Tundra

  Special K
  Stonehedge
  Yumboldt
Sensi Seed Bank
  Big Bud
  Black Domina
  California Indica
  Hash Plant
  Jack Herer
  Northern Lights
  Northern Lights-Haze
  Shiva Skunk
  Silver Pearl
  Super Skunk
Serious Seeds
  AK-47
  Bubble Gum
  Chronic
  Kali Mist
  White Russian
Shadow Seed Co.
  Willy Jack Brainer
Soma's Seeds
  Buddha's Sister
  Kahuna
  Lavender
  Reclining Buddha
  Soma A+
  Somango
TH Seeds
  Chocolate Chunk
  SAGE

aeroponics-growing plants by misting roots suspended in air

apical tip- the growing tip of the plant

backcrossing- crossing of an offspring with one of the parents to reinforce a trait

bract- small reduced leaflet in cannabis that appears below a pair of calyxes

calyx- pod harboring the female ovule and two pistils; seed pod

CBC- cannabichromene. One of several cannabinoids which interact with THC to alter its effects. CBC is non-psychoactive alone

CBD- cannabidiol. One of several cannabinoids which interact with THC to alter its effects. This one makes you sleepy and relaxed, but is not psychoactive

cotyledon- the first pair of leaves of a seed plant

f1 generation- first filial generation, the offspring of two parent (P-1) plants

f2 generation- second filial generation, the offspring of two f1 plants

hydroponics- growing plants in nutrient solution without soil

indica- plant originating in the 30th parallel typified by wide, dark green leaves sometimes bordering on purple. Short internodes and profuse branching form a wide pyramid shape usually no more than $3\frac{1}{2}$ feet tall

internodes- the space between nodes

node- a section of the stem where leaves and side shoots arise. Nodes are often swollen, and are sometimes referred to as joints

P-1- first parental generation, the parents that are crossed to form f1 or f1-hybrid offspring

petiole- the stem of the leaf. It attaches to the plant stem

pistils- small pair of fuzzy, white hairs extending from top of calyx; the flower's female organ

pollen- the male reproductive product that fertilizes the female flower. It is a cream-colored or yellow dust released by the male flower. Cannabis pollen floats along air currents

psychoactive- affecting the consciousness or psyche

radicle- the root of a germinating seed

sativa- plant originating from the 45-50th parallel typified by a tall pine-tree-like growth habit (5 to 15 feet), long internodes, light green color and airy buds

sea of green (SOG)- indoor method for growing marijuana. Many plants are grown close together with little time spent in vegetative growth. Rather than a few plants growing large and filling the canopy, many smaller plants are forced into flowering, creating a lower canopy and earlier harvest

sepal- a modified leaf located at the base of a flower

stigma- the two "hairs" sticking up from each marijuana flower. When young they are white or cream-colored although they sometime have purple tints. They mine the air for pollen. When pollinated or stale they dry and turn tan, red or purple

stipule- the section where the plant stem meets the leaf stem, or petiole

strain- a line of offspring derived from common ancestors

THC- tetrahydrocannabinol. The primary psychoactive component of cannabis

trichome- plant hair that is either glandular (secreting) or eglandular (non-secreting) in function

wpf- watts per square foot

wpm- watts per square meter

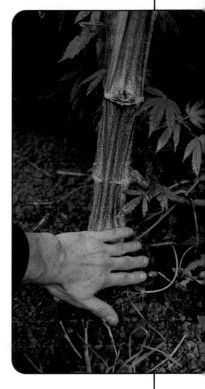

Cannabis flowers based on the number of hours of uninterrupted dark period it receives. When a critical period is reached for several days, the plant changes its growth from vegetative to flowering. During the spring and summer, the number of hours of darkness shrinks as the latitude increases. For instance, June 16, is close to summer solstice (June 22), the longest day of the year and the first day of summer. On June 16 there are $9\frac{1}{2}$ hours (9:30) of darkness at the 35th latitude, near Memphis, Albuquerque and Los Angeles. At the 40th parallel, close to New York, Columbus and Denver the dark period is 9 hours, a difference of a half-hour. However, the seed producers' latitudes are considerably different than the latitudes of the gardens of many outdoor growers. Vancouver, at the 50th parallel and Holland at the 52nd parallel have 7:49 and 7:27 of darkness respectively on that date. As a result, maturity dates change significantly with changes in latitude.

To find the ripening date at your latitude:

1.) Count back from the outdoor ripening date, the days the variety takes to flower indoors. This is the trigger date, the date that the plant changes from vegetative to flowering phase.

2.) Locate the breeder's latitude at the trigger date. The chart indicates the number of hours of darkness at that latitude when the plant was triggered to flower.

3.) In the column representing your latitude, locate the date on the chart that matches the dark period from #2.

4.) Count forward the number of days it takes to ripen indoors. The result is the maturity date.

Figuring Ripening Dates: Examples

A variety from Holland ripens there in mid-October (@ Oct 15) and matures in 70 days indoors. Counting back on the latitude chart you see that on August 1, about 75 days before ripening, the plant triggered on $8\frac{1}{2}$ hours of darkness. Along the 40th parallel or further south, the dark period never gets below 9 hours of darkness. The variety will be triggered to flower almost as soon as it is placed outside. If it's planted outdoors June 1 it will ripen in 70 days, near August 10. If planted June 16 it will ripen in late August. At the 45th parallel, the plant will be triggered to flower around July 1. The buds will mature September 10-15.

A Canadian variety adapted to the 50th parallel ripens October 16 outdoors and 60 days after forcing indoors. Counting back to August 16, 60 days before the bud matures, the dark period at the 50th parallel is about $9\frac{1}{2}$ hours. At the 45th parallel this dark period occurs August 4, with a ripening date of around October 4. At the 40th parallel it occurs around July 30, with a harvest around September 30. At the 35th parallel and lower latitudes, flowering is triggered as soon as the plants are planted since there are only a few days around June 22 when the dark period stretches longer than $9\frac{1}{2}$ hours. If planted June 1, the plants will ripen in early August.

Translating Norhern and Southern Latitudes
The dates listed in the chart below are for Northern latitudes. To figure dates from or for Southern latitudes, add 6 months to the dates that appear. For instance, Aug 1 in the Northern latitudes is equivalent to Feb 1 in Southern latitudes. Seeds from Southern latitudes will mature at the usual fall times in the Northern hemisphere.

NUMBER OF HOURS OF DARKNESS BY LATITUDE												
Latitude	0	+10	+20	+30	+35	+40	+45	+50	+52	+54	+56	+58
June 16	11:53	11:18	10:40	9:56	9:30	8:59	8:24	7:49	7:27	6:53	6:25	5:53
July 1	11:53	11:18	10:41	9:57	9:31	9:01	8:26	7:41	7:21	6:57	6:29	5:55
July 16	11:53	11:21	10:46	10:08	9:44	9:17	8:45	8:05	7:47	7:25	7:01	7:33
Aug 1	11:53	11:27	10:59	10:26	10:06	9:44	9:19	8:48	8:32	8:15	7:57	7:35
Aug 16	11:53	11:34	11:13	10:48	10:33	10:17	9:58	9:35	9:27	9:12	9:59	9:43
Sep 1	11:53	11:42	11:29	11:15	11:06	10:57	10:45	10:29	10.25	10:18	10:10	10:02
Sep 16	11:53	11:50	11:46	11:41	11:39	11:35	11:31	11:27	11:24	11:22	11:21	11:16
Oct 1	11:53	11:59	12:03	12:08	12:11	12:14	12:18	12:22	12:24	12:26	12:28	12:30
Oct 16	11:53	12:07	12:19	12:35	12:43	12:53	13:06	13:17	13:23	13:30	13:36	13:45
Nov 1	11:53	12:13	12:36	13:01	13:15	13:31	13:49	14:14	14:24	14:35	14:48	15:03
Nov 16	11:53	12:21	12:50	13:22	13:42	14:03	14:29	15:00	15:14	15:30	15:49	16:09
Dec 1	11:53	12:26	13:00	13:39	14:03	14:27	14:58	15:36	16:07	16:14	16:36	17:02
Dec 16	11:53	12:27	13:05	13:56	14:12	14:40	15:12	15:54	16:13	16:36	17:01	17:31

Breeder Latitudes:

Australia: Nimbin: Latitude 30 S
Canada: Ottawa-Toronto, Ontario: Latitude 43 N
         Vancouver, British Columbia: Latitude 50 N
Holland: Latitude 52 N
Malawi: Latitudes 10-15 S
Swaziland: Latitude 26 S
Switzerland: Latitude: 47 N

METRIC CONVERSION

Mass

1 gram = .035 ounces (1/3 ounce)
1 ounce = 28.35 grams
1 pound = 16 ounces
1 kilogram = 2.20 pounds
1 lb. = .45 kilograms (about 1/2 kilogram)

Length

1 foot = .30 meters
1 meter = 3.28 feet
1 meter = 100 centimeters
1 inch = 2.54 centimeters

Area

1 square meter = 10.76 square feet
1 square foot = .09 square meters

Yield

1 ounce per f2 = 305 g per m2
100 g per m2 = 3.25 ounces per f2

Temperature

Celsius to Fahrenheit
15 C = 59 F
20 C = 68 F
22 C = 72 F
25 C = 77 F
28 C = 82 F
30 C = 86 F
32 C = 89.5 F
35 C = 95 F
To figure:
Celsius = (F - 32) * 5/9
Fahrenheit = C * 9/5 + 32

Blue Velvet
Bubbleberry
Bubble Gum
Chronic
Critical Mass
Dutch Dragon
Early Queen
Eclipse
Flo
Hashmaster
Hawaiian Haze
Ice
Island Sweet Skunk
Jack Herer
Kahuna
La Niña
Lavender
Léda Uno
Max 49
Medicine Man
Nebula
Nevil's Haze
Niagara
Niagara x Shiva
Northern Lights-Haze
The Pure Skunk #1
The Real McCoy
SAGE
Silver Haze
Somango
Special Haze
Special K
Spice
Super Silver Haze

Super Skunk
Ultra Skunk
White Shark
White Widow

 S **sativa strains (81–100% sativa)**
Hawaiian Sativa
Kali Mist
Malawi Gold
New Purple Power
Old Mother Sativa
Swazi Safari
Swazi Skunk

Varieties by Indoor & Outdoor
Note that category may be in part determined by area of origin. See the variety's description for more detailed information.

 indoor strains
Betazoid
Big Bud
Black Domina
Blueberry x Nice
Bubble Gum
Caramella
Eclipse
Hash Plant
Hawaiian Haze
Haze 19 x Skunk #1
Ice
Jack Herer
Master Kush
Misty

Northern Lights
Northern Lights-Haze
Original Misty
Pot of Gold
Shiva Skunk
Silver Blue
Silver Pearl
Super Skunk
White Russian
Willy Jack Brainer

 indoor/outdoor strains

AK-47
Americano
Amsterdam Flame
Atomic Northern Lights
BC Big Bud
Belladonna
Black Widow
Blueberry
Blueberry x Northern Lights
Blue Moonshine
Blue Skunk Special
Blue Velvet
Bubbleberry
Buddha's Sister
California Indica
Chocolate Chunk
Chronic
Critical Mass
Devil
Durga Mata
Dutch Dragon
Dutchmen's Royal Orange

Early Queen
El Niño
Flo
Hashmaster
Hawaiian Sativa
Island Sweet Skunk
Kahuna
Kali Mist
KC 33
La Niña
Lavender
Léda Uno
Mango
Mangolian Indica
Matanuska Tundra
Max 49
Medicine Man
Millennium
Nebula
Nevil's Haze
Niagara
Niagara x Shiva
Northern Lights x Bubble Gum
The Pure Skunk #1
The Real McCoy
Reclining Buddha
Romulan
SAGE
Sensi Star
Shark Shock
Sheherazade
Shit
Silver Haze
Soma A+

Somango
Special Haze
Special K
Spice
Stonehedge
Super Silver Haze
Swazi Safari
Swazi Skunk
Ultra Skunk
White KC
White Shark
White Widow
Yumboldt

 outdoor strains
Bahia Black Head
Huron
Malawi Gold
Mikado
New Purple Power
Old Mother Sativa
Sweet Purple

Greenhouse Varieties

While many all-around strains can perform well in the greenhouse, the following strains were particularly noted by the breeders as appropriate for greenhouse cultivation.

Blue Skunk Special
California Indica
Devil
Dutchmen's Royal Orange
Flo

New Purple Power
The Pure Skunk #1
The Real McCoy
Shit
Super Skunk

Sea of Green Varieties

While other strains may also work in a sea of green growing method, breeders have named the following varieties as most conducive to this method.

Atomic Northern Lights
BC Big Bud
Belladonna
Big Bud
Black Domina
Blueberry
Blueberry x Nice
Blue Velvet
Bubbleberry
Bubble Gum
Chronic
Durga Mata
Dutch Dragon
Early Queen
Eclipse
Hashmaster
Hash Plant
Hawaiian Sativa
Ice
Island Sweet Skunk
Kahuna
Kali Mist

Essays, Stories & Illustrations

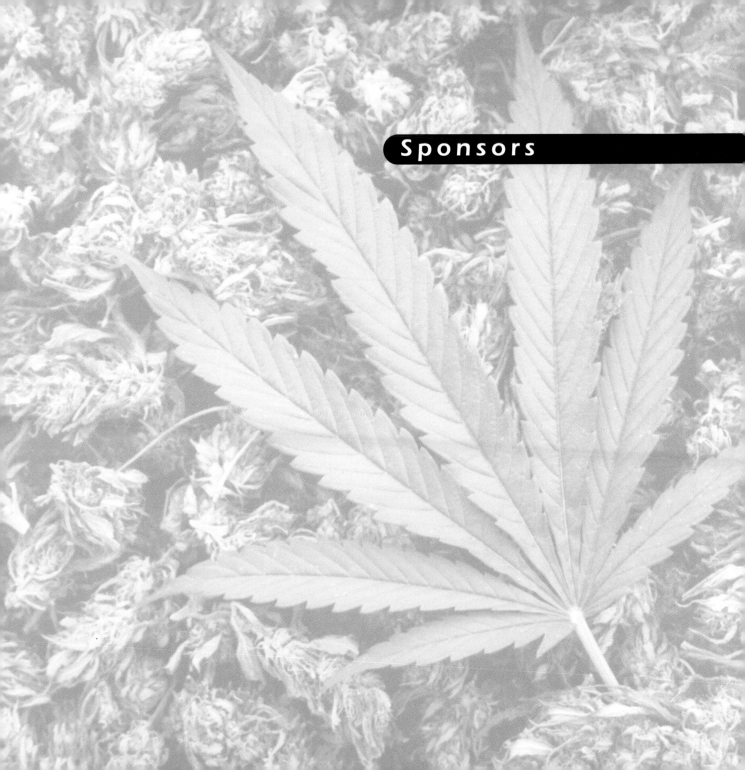

Sponsors

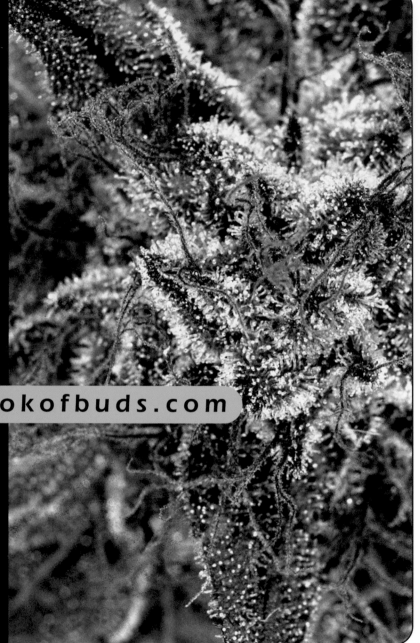

The Big Book of
BUDS

thanks the
businesses that
supported this
project.

Online photo
gallery of the
best marijuana
in the world.

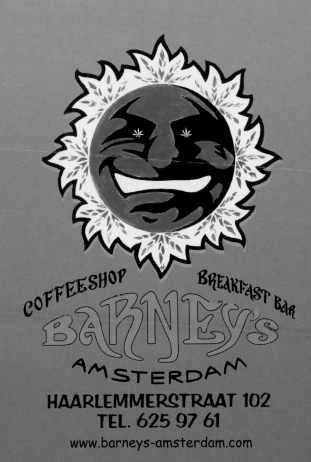

COFFEESHOP   BREAKFAST BAR

BARNEY's

AMSTERDAM

HAARLEMMERSTRAAT 102
TEL. 625 97 61

www.barneys-amsterdam.com

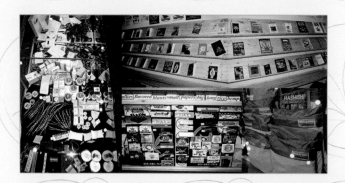
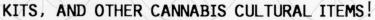
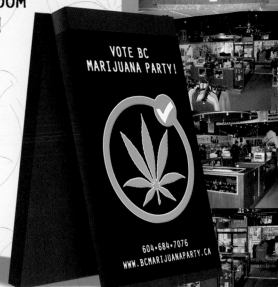

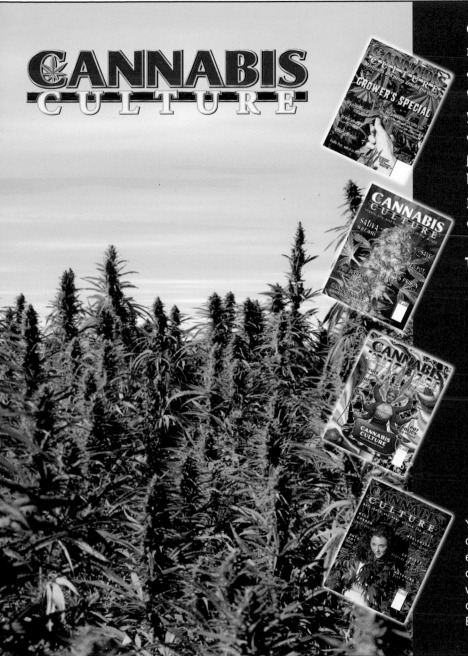

201

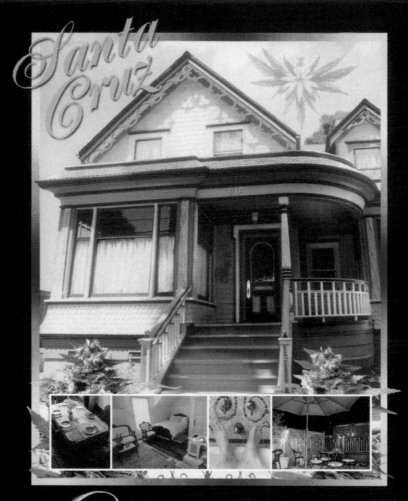

Santa Cruz

Compassion Flower Inn

A bed, bud and breakfast serving the medical marijuana community and all world travelers who honor the many uses of the hemp plant.

216 Laurel Street, Santa Cruz, California 95060 / phone 831 466-0420

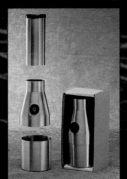
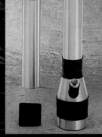
203

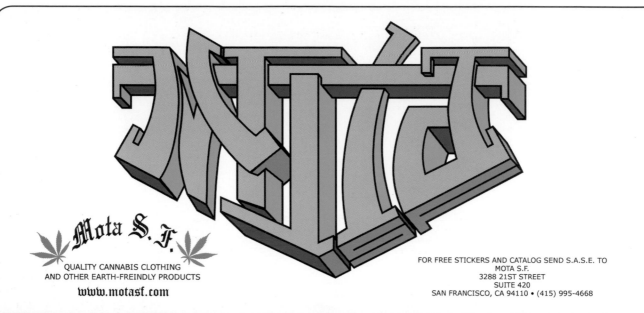
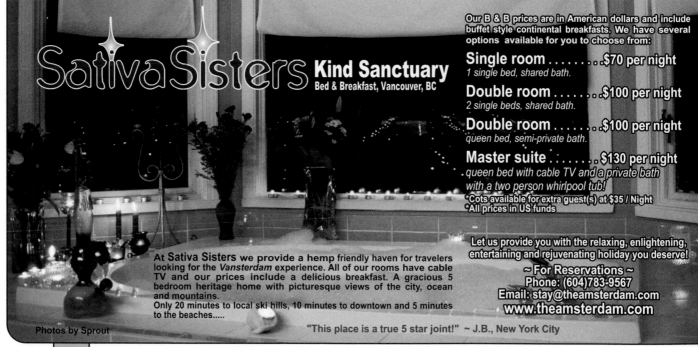

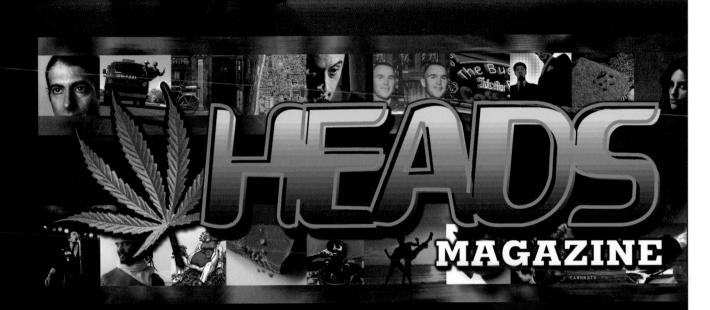

HEADS MAGAZINE

It's a state of mind

www.headsmagazine.com

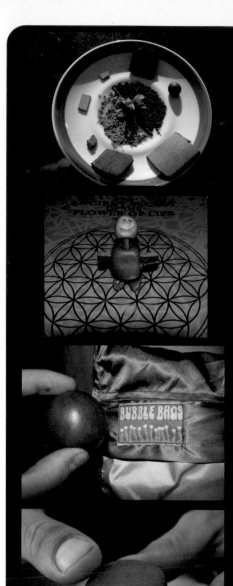

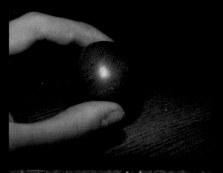

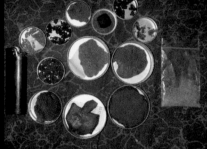

Bubble Bags
The Perfect Tool for Harvesting Your Freshest Headies

Visit our website to learn more about
Bubble Bags
and
Cold Water Hash Extraction
www.bubblebag.com

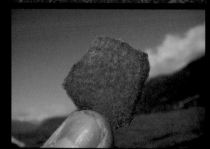

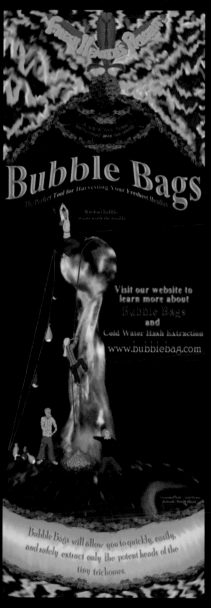

Bubble Bags will allow you to quickly, easily, and safely extract only the potent heads of the tiny trichomes.

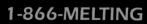

1-866-MELTING

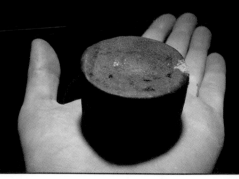

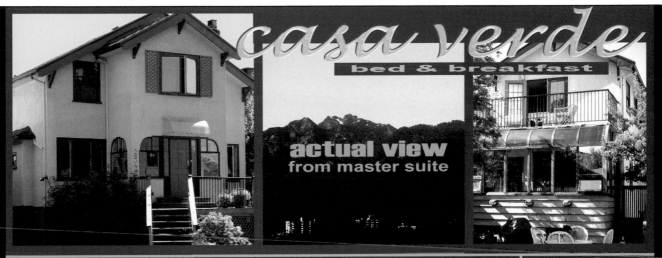
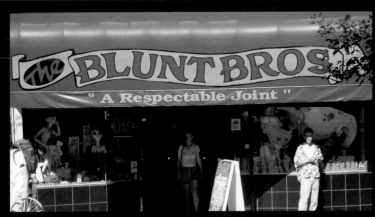
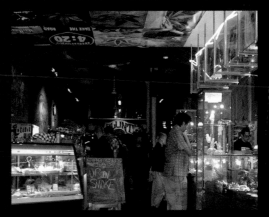
207

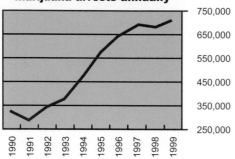
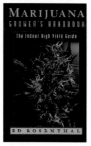
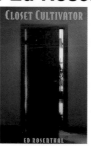
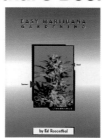
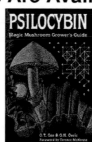
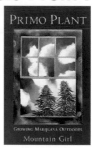
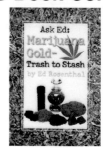

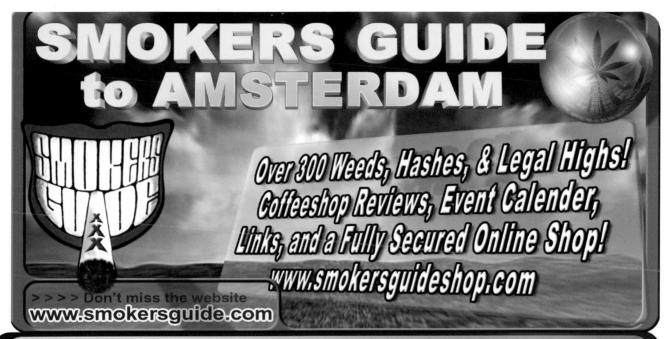
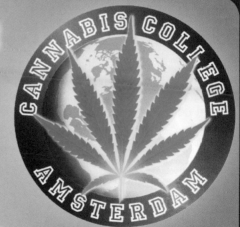

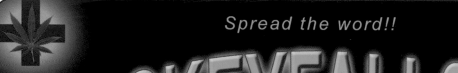
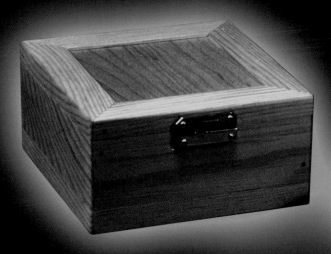
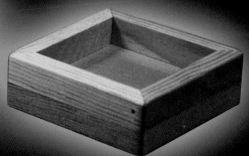

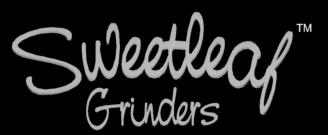
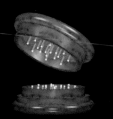
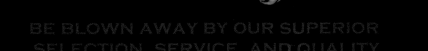

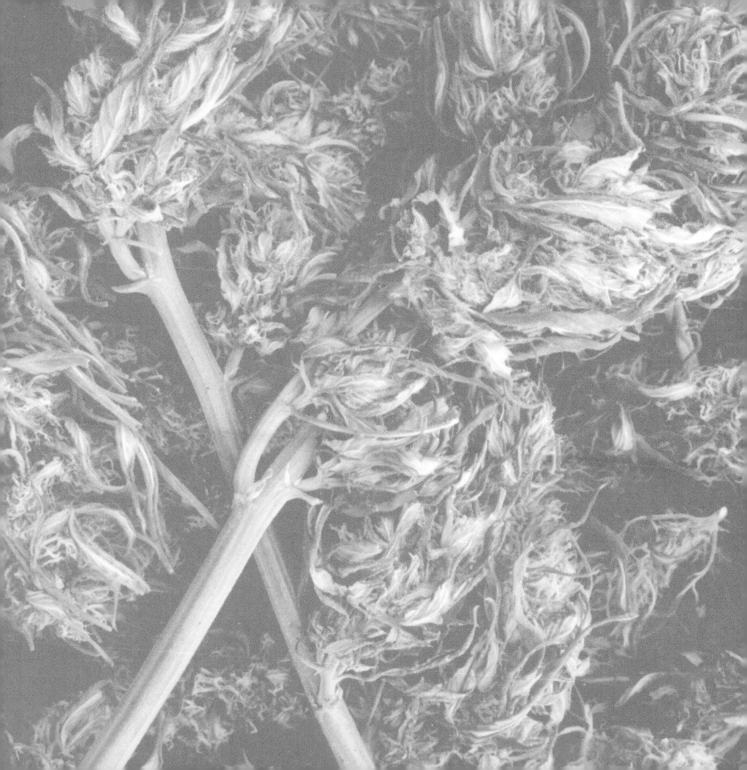

Quick Key to Icons

English ▪ En Español ▪ Deutsch
En Français ▪ Italiano ▪ Dutch

Strain Type

Sativa   Indica   Sativa/Indica   Indica/Sativa

Growing Info

               SOG

Flowering time	Parents	Yield	Sea of
Tiempo de floración	Genética	Rendimiento	Green
Blütezeit	Mutterpflanze	Ertag	
Durée de floraison	Descendance	Rendement	
Stagione della	Genitori	Raccolta	
fioritura ▪ Bloeitijd	Stamboom	Opbrengst	

Indoor ▪ Interior   Outdoor ▪ Exterior   Indoor/Outdoor
Drinnen ▪ d'Intérieur   Draussen ▪ d'Extérieur
Dentro ▪ Binnen   Fuori ▪ Buiten

Sensory Experience

Buzz ▪ Efecto   Taste/Smell ▪ Sabor/Aroma
die Art des Turns   Geschmack/Geruch
Effets ▪ Effetti   Saveur/Arôme
High Effekt   Sapore/Odore ▪ Smaak/Geua

Grower Location

South Africa   Australia   Canada

Netherlands   Switzerland